INTRODUCTION TO KEY CONCEPTS AND EVOLUTIONS IN PSYCHOANALYSIS

Introduction to Key Concepts and Evolutions in Psychoanalysis offers an accessible starting point to understanding psychoanalysis by focusing on seven key psychoanalytic models and their creators and how the field has evolved over time from Sigmund Freud's original ideas. The book is based on the premise that Freud started a conversation over 100 years ago that continues to this day: who are we, why do we suffer so, and how can others help?

Alexis A. Johnson seeks to make the invariably complex and sometimes contradictory terms and concepts of psychoanalysis more accessible for those being introduced to psychoanalysis for the first time, integrating them into a cohesive narrative, while using a broadly developmental perspective. Each model is given space and context, matched with relevant case studies drawn from the author's own clinical practice.

Written in an approachable, jargon-free style, this book brings to life the creators of the models using case studies to illustrate the 'healing maps' and models they have developed. The author methodically adds layer upon layer of increasingly challenging insights: Which model is useful or appropriate, and when and how exactly is it useful as part of the healing paradigm? Rather than aligning with any one model, Johnson makes the case that drawing upon aspects of all of these sometimes-competing ideas at various times is important and healthy.

Introduction to Key Concepts and Evolutions in Psychoanalysis will appeal to undergraduate students of psychology encountering psychoanalysis for the first time, as well as trainees in psychoanalysis and those working across other branches of the mental health profession wishing to understand and draw upon fundamental psychoanalytic ideas.

Alexis A. Johnson has been in private practice as a clinical psychologist in the Greater New York City area for nearly 50 years. She also is Co-Director of the Center for Intentional Living.

INTRODUCTION TO KEY CONCEPTS AND EVOLUTIONS IN PSYCHOANALYSIS

From Freud to Neuroscience

Alexis A. Johnson

Routledge
Taylor & Francis Group
LONDON AND NEW YORK

First published 2019
by Routledge
2 Park Square, Milton Park, Abingdon, Oxon OX14 4RN

and by Routledge
52 Vanderbilt Avenue, New York, NY 10017

Routledge is an imprint of the Taylor & Francis Group, an informa business

British Library Cataloguing in Publication Data
A catalogue record for this book is available from the British Library

Library of Congress Cataloging in Publication Data
Names: Johnson, Alexis A., 1944- author.
Title: Introduction to key concepts and evolutions in psychoanalysis : from Freud to neuroscience / Alexis A. Johnson.
Description: New York : Routledge, 2019. | Includes bibliographical references and index.
Identifiers: LCCN 2018036224 (print) | LCCN 2018041229 (ebook) | ISBN 9780429467301 (Master) | ISBN 9780429884238 (Web PDF) | ISBN 9780429884221 (ePub) | ISBN 9780429884214 (Mobipocket/Kindle) | ISBN 9781138607125 (hardback : alk. paper) | ISBN 9781138607132 (pbk. : alk. paper)
Subjects: LCSH: Psychoanalysis—History.
Classification: LCC BF173 (ebook) | LCC BF173 .J544 2019 (print) | DDC 150.19/5—dc23
LC record available at https://lccn.loc.gov/2018036224

ISBN: 978-1-138-60712-5 (hbk)
ISBN: 978-1-138-60713-2 (pbk)
ISBN: 978-0-429-46730-1 (ebk)

Typeset in Bembo
by Swales & Willis Ltd, Exeter, Devon, UK

For my cherished students and for seekers everywhere—
the askers of challenging questions, the pioneers of healing conversations

CONTENTS

Acknowledgments *viii*

Introduction 1

1 Sigmund Freud: we are all in inner conflict 4

2 The bridge between Freud and modern psychoanalysis 21

3 Melanie Klein: life is terrifying, and we must survive 26

4 Anna Freud: we have strengths as well as conflicts 48

5 The middle school: with good enough mothering, we evolve from ruthless to "ruth" 64

6 Heinz Kohut: we always need others for our well-being and to create meaning 88

7 Harry Sullivan: we need relationships to manage our anxieties and to thrive 107

8 John Bowlby: lost connection is traumatic; secure attachment is the key to well-being 125

9 Emergent complexity: Freud to neuroscience 147

Glossary *163*

Index *176*

ACKNOWLEDGMENTS

First and foremost, I wish to thank the fabulous team at Routledge, especially Charles Bath, Kate Hawes, Rosie Stewart, Graham Frankland, and others, who helped to bring this book to life and answered every question with patience and enthusiasm. I am forever grateful for your guidance.

As anyone knows, it takes many minds to create a book. Among those who have helped me the most are my friend and colleague of 40 years, Judith Schmidt, with her constant intellectual and emotional inspiration; Sandy Cotter, another persistent voice, who also read and reacted to every line with enormous love and attention; my editor, Lia Dangelico, with her fine attention to detail, constant support, and excellent feedback; and my husband, Jerome Kerner, without whom I would not be the person I am today. An extra heap of gratitude to Jerome for the beautiful illustrations he sketched to accompany each chapter of this book. Thank you.

INTRODUCTION

I consider myself a humanistic psychologist, having fallen in love with the ideas of Abraham Maslow, Carl Rogers, and Martin Buber many years ago. This powerful movement championed our innate capacity for growth and change. Maslow told us of self-actualization and peak experiences. Rogers taught unconditional positive regard, and Buber wrote that all human interaction needs to reach for the ideal of an "I" with a "thou." I still hold these principles as my inner bedrock. They are my ideals, my aspirations.

However, when sitting with the people who have come my way—whether they are called patients or clients—I also have found that I need a more in-depth understanding of mind and motivation, change and healing than the humanistic tradition offers me. The British and American psychoanalytic traditions, all in various conversations with the founding father Sigmund Freud, have provided me the frameworks needed to be with the suffering that enters my consulting room. I have needed both Freud himself and these thinkers in order to formulate my own questions to open the deep feelings and fantasies that underpin my clients' defenses and issues. In the psychoanalytic tradition, there are vivid models of how people experience their ever-changing senses of self, as well as guidance as to how I might enter their reality enough to be a companion on the journey. These maps also help me understand and appreciate myself in my complexity, reactions, feelings, and moods. As I studied and worked with these various traditions, I found that the big thinkers disagree profoundly and often. I have come to hold these discrepancies lightly, finding a better fit for some clients in one model and for some in another. As a result, each of these models now has a place in my thinking. I am making no attempt to criticize these analysts nor explicate their work in any complete way; rather, I am drawing upon concepts from each of them that I have found valuable and useful.

For the last 40 years, I have been teaching various aspects of psychotherapy to eclectic therapists, like myself, and to other interested professionals. Over the past 18 years, I have been particularly blessed with an intellectual community based in England that likes to gather twice a year for an intensive, three-day seminar. This group includes psychotherapists, executive coaches, and human resources professionals, all of whom are too busy to read up on all they would like to know about psychology. So, every six months, we decide on a topic to explore and I have the delight of plunging into research followed by the pleasure of sharing what I have learned with them. Together, we discuss, process, discover, and grow. We have explored a wide range of topics, including the foundations of psychotherapy, family systems, fatherhood, bereavement and death, betrayal and lust, spiritual awareness and the nature of consciousness, and many more. We have discussed everything from Wilhelm Reich's ideas about sexuality and orgone energy, to Donald Winnicott's transitional objects and Ken Wilber's integral theory, to current neuroscience and the usefulness of mindfulness.

This book is built around one of those three-day seminars. I was asked by several members of the group to tell the human and philosophical story of the evolution of psychoanalytic thinking. "How did we get where we are?" I have picked the thinkers who most influenced my clinical work and told the story of how they fit together in my mind. This is not a complete story in any sense; in fact, it is closer to the tip of an iceberg. However, these are people and ideas that I have found to be crucial to my work with patients and understanding people in general. This book also is an invitation and a resource for other intellectually curious people.

In this book, I narrate the evolution of Freud's original theories and contributions to modern psychotherapy. After all, it is a story; it is one way of looking at the last 150 years of psychological development with an eye to both understanding oneself and helping others. My own style of learning is to move between primary and secondary sources to elucidate a clinical issue or a question that has come up in a seminar. I enjoy knowing how other minds have looked at the issues originally conceptualized by the "old masters." I have tried to present key concepts in as clear and relevant a fashion as I can, knowing that many nuances and specifics have to be left out in order to stay true to that intent.

Each contributor to the field of psychoanalysis had a personal predilection, based on his or her personal history and influenced by the times in which he or she lived. Thus, Freud wanted to create an objective natural science, as that was critical in his time. As a displaced European Jew living in Chicago, Heinz Kohut was looking for meaning and mattering. Harry Stack Sullivan saw anxiety everywhere, as that was his personal experience. These personal circumstances and predilections are an important part of my understanding this history.

The following is my way of using the innovations contributed by the major schools of modern-day psychoanalysis in the United States and England. I have divided them into six lines of thought, accepting that, today, many individuals belong to more than one lineage. The Kleinian school, the ego psychologists, and the British middle school all started their conversations by the 1930s in London.

The self psychology and relational school came later in the United States. Interestingly, John Bowlby, with the power of his attachment theory, was part of that first British world, but was accepted in the United States before he was acknowledged in England. Together, these six traditions elucidate, consolidate, and evolve Freud's first paradigm-breaking ideas.

One final and important note: For the sake of privacy, all of the patient stories I present here are amalgams of the many people I have sat with over the years. However, I intend to convey the emotional truth of these encounters with each of my illustrations.

Freud's lineage

Drive	*Ego*	*Middle school*	*Self*	*Interpersonal relationship*	*Attachment*
Klein (1882–1960)	A. Freud (1895–1982)	Fairbairn (1889–1964)	Kohut (1913–81)	Sullivan (1892–1949)	Bowlby (1907–90)
Bion (1897–1979)	Hartmann (1894–1970)	Balint (1896–1970)	Stolorow & Atwood	Fromm (1900–80)	Ainsworth (1913–99)
Kernberg	Spitz (1887–1974)	Winnicott (1896–1971)	Brandchaft (1916–2013)	Thompson (1893–1958)	Main
Ogden	Mahler (1897–1985)	Guntrip (1901–75)	Stern (1932–2012)	Aron	Fonagy
	Erikson (1902–94)	Bollas	Beebe & Lachmann	Mitchell (1946–2000)	Schore
			Orange	Bromberg	Siegel
					Porges

1

SIGMUND FREUD

We are all in inner conflict

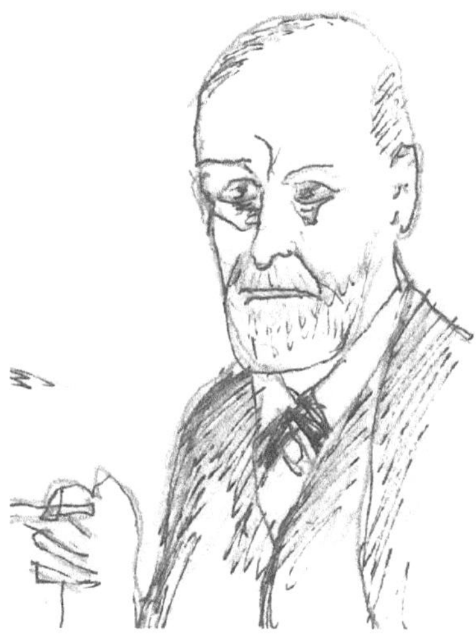

Sigmund Freud

From the position of over a century later, we can see that Sigmund Freud (1856–1939) transformed Western culture and sensibility. He changed forever how we think about others and ourselves. He wrote about all things human: sexuality, sadism, masochism, love, jealousy, cruelty, curiosity, and wit (Bloom, 1986). Charles Darwin (1809–1882) had already placed human beings squarely in the animal kingdom. Freud concurred with Darwin: We are biological creatures, driven by instincts, and pushed by unknown forces from within our own selves. He saw us as originating from biological givens with a body and a mind and wanted his intellectual contributions to be in the realm of science. By modern standards, he was not a scientist, he was a theorizer, even a myth-maker. Like each of us, he was a product of his time and was writing in the context in which he found himself, politically, socially, and scientifically. Body and mind were considered separate parts of human beings, and as a neurologist he was interested in how they interacted. What part of the brain creates the mind, that specific sense of self that each of us calls "me?" Freud realized that he did not have the tools to literally look into the brain and discover its workings, but he believed he could discern how the mind worked by listening and observing deeply.

Freud pointed us in many new directions. He maintained that the invisible workings of both the mind and the emotions were vital and capable of being studied. He firmly believed that we could come to understand our human minds without direct physical observations. As therapists, we would need to *interpret* what can be seen and heard in order to infer the workings of the mind and emotions (Freud, 1900; 1917b). In short, he was confident that we could know the inner, the invisible.

Today, most therapists and counselors don't seem to think they need to study Freud, as much of our understanding of the human mind and its diseases and discomforts has evolved in other directions. We have medical models that think in terms of biochemical and neuronal connections. We have object-relations theory and attachment theory. We have learning theories and systems theory. All of these provide a very different understanding of the human mind than the classical Freudian model.

However, I believe we need to have at least a passing familiarity with Freud to be both a member of Western culture and a therapist interested in depth and complexity. We have to know what the "Freudian slip" refers to if we are going to have some insight regarding how we undermine ourselves in everyday life or catch others in an unguarded moment. What if we couldn't get the well-known Freudian joke: "A psychotic thinks two and two are five. A neurotic knows two and two are four and hates it." What a loss that would be! (Freud, 1901; Freud, A., 1935)

Harold Bloom (1986) remarked that psychoanalysis has become a tiny branch in psychiatry, but that Freud himself is the greatest myth-maker of the last century, and disciplines from history to literary criticism can and do use aspects of his remarkable body of work. Because of Freud's impact, we all automatically think psychologically in Western society; that is, we "know" that humans are complex and conflicted and often don't understand themselves. Each of us is a house divided against itself. We look for motives and understanding in art, education, literature, movies, all of the social sciences, and more. Freud's lexicon is part of our everyday conversations. We recognize that the "anal" person hoards or is tight with money or feelings or words. We call the smoker an "oral" or say he has an "oral fixation." We know that "libido" refers to our ongoing interest in sex and all things sexual. And, finally, we know that Woody Allen is neurotic, not just because he tells us so. We know what "neurotic" means without being told—these words have become part of our everyday language.

Even though many of the Freudian specifics have been rejected both by modern psychoanalysis and psychotherapy, so much has been incorporated into modern thinking that we do not even recognize it as coming from Freud. It just is. We accept that we have a conscious and an unconscious. We accept that we have various defenses: we "project," we "deny," we "sublimate." We admit that sexuality and aggression are very powerful, non-rational, and often get us into a lot of trouble. Moreover, all of our self-help groups operate on the premise that emotional talking is somehow helpful, somehow gets us out of ruts, out of being stuck. Most of us believe that change is possible, that we can understand ourselves and, therefore, help ourselves live more fulfilling lives. Thank you, Professor Freud.

Freud influenced modern life profoundly and continues to influence aspects of intellectual life today. At the same time, the specifics of his thinking have been radically altered, some beyond recognition. These are my understandings of this lineage—how it has affected modern thinking about the mind and the psyche, and what it means to be human. I have chosen to highlight the concepts he gave us that have most helped me in my clinical practice, even if some of them have been greatly modified by modern information.

Trauma

Freud was following in the footsteps of two other men who were deeply interested in helping people suffering from the psychological pain called "hysteria," Josef Breuer (1842–1925) and Jean-Martin Charcot (1825–1893). In the late 19th century, men in general and doctors in particular "knew" that women had mysterious emotional events that overwhelmed them and rendered them irrational, unable to express what was happening to them in an orderly and systematic way. This term, "hysteria," derives from the Greek as coming "from the womb." Hysteria was a focus of scientific inquiry even though it was not defined in any specific way. Rather, it was a somewhat puzzling group of symptoms: seizures of unknown origin, an inability to speak, strange paralyses that did not make sense given known neurology, and the occasional hallucination. Scientists had pieced together the idea that if they could trace the sufferer's words back in time, they would find an original event, the root of the suffering. They noted that simply knowing the root usually was not sufficient. The sufferer needed both the knowledge and, simultaneously, a strong emotional discharge coming out of that knowledge, called the abreaction. This combination of bringing the root cause into awareness and experiencing the pain, upset, and rage that the event engendered seemed to allow the symptoms to alleviate and, sometimes, disappear altogether. (Today in cases of PTSD, whether by sexual trauma or war trauma, this combination is still helpful in some instances.)

In 1896, Freud published "The aetiology of hysteria." This paper proposed that the symptoms of hysteria were caused by trapped memories of premature sexual experience, which were stored in an altered state of consciousness where such memories were not "remembered" or "understood." These disconnected memories were stored away from the conscious self and were typically of a character that would be unacceptable to the everyday sense of self. In this way, Freud gave us the first in-depth understanding of "trauma," as well as "dissociation" and "traumatic memory." Nearly a century of evolving understanding would pass before we had a fuller and deeper picture of mind, memory, and trauma. Only now can we fully appreciate the power of these unremembered yet unforgotten memories (Herman, 1992).

Freud's original theory of the causes of hysteria involved trauma, what we would now call "relational" or "developmental" or "sexual" trauma. In their past, bad things had happened to the women suffering from these highly disorganizing and distressing symptoms. These upsetting events had been at least partially forgotten or "repressed," to use another Freudian term. They could not be faced or talked about and, as a result, daily life was impacted by their disruptive and distressing manifestations. Freud's first belief was that it was the premature forced introduction to sexuality that caused the symptoms of hysteria. Young women reported instances of sexual violation from family or friends, or incest at the hands of family members. But the idea that such things had concretely happened—that young girls had been molested or were victims of incest—was not admissible to him or his times. He turned away from the disturbing data he was uncovering in his study of the origin of hysterical symptoms (Herman, 1992).

Within the following year, Freud repudiated his initial thesis that hysteria was caused by trauma and, specifically, infantile or early sexual trauma. His mind could not hold the idea that this much sexual abuse was happening in his Viennese world, and he could not expect to become a recognized success if he brought forth such shocking information. Faced with this dilemma, Freud sought to generate a new theory. In a sense, he stopped listening to the women he so carefully documented in 1896. Instead, he created a new theory based on an inner life of fantasy and imagination, espousing that the source of the problem lay within the women themselves, not their environment. Rather than being exploited and seduced by adults, hysterical women were seen as having created sexual, wish-fulfilling fantasies that needed to be repressed (Freud, 1905). It is important to note that, at this time, it was assumed by men that only men had sexual urges and that a woman was a delicate creature, who required only protection and the gift of children in order to have a fulfilled life. Overall, 19th-century Victorian culture refused to admit the possibility of sexual abuse.

Due to these conflicts and discrepancies, the whole enterprise of studying hysteria melted away during the following decade, and the content and focus of psychoanalysis changed. Freud and his followers became interested in other aspects of psychoanalysis: various forms of neurotic suffering, the nature of dreams, the technique of "free association," and what became called "transference" within the doctor–patient dyad. The creation of theory and technique became paradoxically both intertwined and disconnected.

The drive-conflict model

In his first attempt to understand his hysterical patients, Freud listened hard to what they were telling him. What he heard astounded him. He heard stories of urges to do forbidden things; he heard about debilitating anxiety, agonizing guilt, and paralyzing inner conflicts. When he repudiated trauma as the cause of these symptoms, he turned to the imagination, concluding that fantasies, wishes, urges, drives, and conflicts must be at the root of the problem.

The drive-conflict model is based on the innate raw power of sensual-sexual pleasures. According to this model, we are each born with urgent needs to be fed, held, and taken care of. These drives are part of what he called our "id," our primitive animal nature. For Freud, our id lives in our unconscious, and at the beginning of life—and for some, for all of life—it is in the driver's seat (Freud, 1905). Its demands are immediate and urgent. For example, when I am hungry, I need to eat now. The id is timeless; that is, it does not recognize the passage of time. The primary id neither recognizes nor tolerates the concept of "later," much less of waiting.

These powerful instincts are both life-affirming and life-denying. Freud divided them into opposing forces: the first being "Eros," which focuses on pleasure and survival. Eros controls the mechanisms for sustaining life, such as respiration, digestion, and, importantly, sexual impulses. Eros is the bonding energy, which enables us to connect first with our parents; later, with lovers; and ultimately, with life itself. He named the energy created by Eros "libido." Libido is the energy of wanting in the positive sense: want of food, pleasure, sexual connection. Eros is life-giving, life-promoting, and life-enriching.

Freud named the opposing force to Eros "Thanatos," meaning our destructive capacities (Freud, 1920). Freud's early faith that human aggression could be contained by psychoanalysis gave way to his belief that human beings are not only aggressive but also cruel and violent. In his later correspondence with Albert Einstein (1932; Einstein, Nathan, & Norden, 1960), he acknowledged his pessimism about humanity given our capacity and appetite for war. Many believe that the pessimistic idea of Thanatos—a wish for death—was born of Freud's own despair after living through World War I, arguably one of the most horrific events in Western history. During this time, he endured the consequences of our human capacity for destruction at the collective level.

Freud shocked his society by suggesting that, within his definition of the pleasure-serving deep vitality of Eros, babies are sexual (Mitchell & Black, 1995; Storr, 1989). I believe what he actually meant was that babies are sensual and pleasure-driven, and that the instinct he named Eros, the life force, operates from the beginning of life. This particular connection was rather crucial at the time because Freud wanted to place psychotherapy and psychoanalysis firmly in the camp of the natural sciences. In order to do this, he needed to link adult sexuality—Darwin's driver of evolution—with some kind of developmental theory. From hours and hours of listening to people, he became increasingly aware of the levels and layers of human complexity and sought to find some way of fitting what psychoanalysis was revealing into the realms of science.

For Freud, discharge is the ultimate pleasure, the goal of the id drives. Freud recognized that, though we are a cauldron of seething impulses, we do not typically boil over into destruction. Some other part of us must moderate those impulses. This moderating aspect he called "ego." The ego in each of us has the tough job of creating a balance between the archaic demands of the id and the reality of the outside world.

In his later thinking, Freud added a third structure to these two, named the "superego." Freud realized that he needed to account for how children internalize their parents' ways and values and ranked the superego as another key internal structure. His notion was that, as the child matured, he or she incorporated what he referred to as the "ego ideal," the standards and values that the child perceives as valuable in his or her family. This combination of id, ego, and superego is the unconscious inner structure that the child carries into adulthood and forms the basis of his personality and defenses.

Freud's superego is an internalized set of rules, standards, and requirements from the outside world that form both our personal family and our wider culture. Together, these three structures influence every aspect of our lives: thoughts, feelings, behaviors, and ideals. At the same time, only the ego is conscious; the id and the superego exert their influence behind closed doors (Brenner, 1955, 1974).

In summary, Freud's early model of a human being included impulses and passions, along with defenses and repression to hold those impulses out of awareness and expression. Freud's drive model started with sexual pleasure-oriented impulses; later managed by the more mature, adult part called the ego; and influenced for better or worse by the superego.

Technique

Free association

When Freud focused on his techniques of healing emotional pain, his first fundamental rule asked his patients to, with absolute honesty, free associate to whatever dreams or thoughts came to mind during the session. Freud's injunction encouraged his patients to relate whatever came to mind, no matter how absurd, trivial, or disagreeable. His hope was that if he stayed personally neutral—out of the way—the patient could find his own words, rather than the words or theories of the doctor—now called "analyst" in this new venture called psychoanalysis. In this way, the patient could begin to examine his own mind and face his own impulses and fantasies. Freud wanted to create a neutral environment, wherein both he and his patient could explore what was going on in the patient's mind. Over time, this method was extended to include reflections from the analyst to encourage the patient to discover and face more of himself. Connections were made. Meaning was created. Very slowly, a more integrated individual emerged as the conflicts and unconscious desires were faced and understood (Mitchell & Black, 1995).

Transference

Freud also noted that his patients often created unconscious assumptions about him—assumptions that stemmed from their own childhood and history with their own parents (Freud, 1912). He was astute enough to note that this unconscious process happened universally, and at first, he thought it was a form of resistance to the basic tool of free association. In due course, he recognized it as a very useful event because it revealed, within the analytic dyad, how the patient related to other people, particularly those they shared intimate relationships with or those in authority. This process, named "transference," revealed in the living moment the fundamental conflicts the patient was trying to resolve. Freud realized that each patient was projecting unconscious childhood expectations and perceptions onto him and then relating to him as if he actually were that other person—usually, their parent.

Today, most all psychoanalysts and most psychotherapists recognize the reality of transference. How it is used differs widely. For me, it is an aspect of the therapeutic relationship that I internally attune to constantly, choosing to talk about it only when I deem it to be helpful. I pay close attention to how a new client first enters my office, as that is an indication of how he or she expects to be received in the world. Individuals will transfer their early feelings of being welcomed or not welcomed on to this new experience of entering my office, meeting a stranger, or starting a new conversation.

When I first met "Jess," she did not look at me directly. She sat on the edge of the couch in my office, appearing very uncomfortable and anxious, trying to figure out what I wanted from her. Jess' mother was very erratic, unpredictable, and sometimes explosive. As a consequence, Jess is almost always on edge when around another woman, especially a woman she sees as an authority, or "in charge" in some way.

"Suzi" presents very differently: She walks in, taking off her jacket as she moves; throws it on a chair; introduces herself; and begins to speak as if we were already in the middle of a conversation. In her family, the center of the universe was her father, and she was his favorite. Suzi not only expects to be welcomed but almost adored, her every word and thought important to all around her.

Both of these women carry their early experiences into the present, as does each of us. Jess and Suzi present to me and to the world very differently yet, out of sight, they both are lonely and long for more human connection in their lives.

Freud regularly experienced that his patients, both men and women, fell in love with him. He called this experience positive transference. I don't believe that Freud used this experience for self-aggrandizement in any way. However, this repetitive experience of positive transference piqued his curiosity. Why, he wondered, would people idealize him as an omnipotent father figure, placing enormous hope in him, and believing he could and would help rid them of their suffering in some magical way? Freud's patients were in deep distress with problems that were invisible to others. They were pained in their minds, not with a broken bone that could be objectively demonstrated to others. They needed him to believe in their stories, to understand their emotions, and to help them find a way through their words into a more integrated, peaceful way of being in the world. Within this context, we can understand why many suffering patients, then and now, forgo a "realistic" view of their therapists, elevating them to near-magical status, desperately hoping for both understanding and a cure for their distress.

Freud also recognized and experienced the opposite phenomena of negative and ambivalent transferences, where the therapist was seen more as a devil figure than an angel. However, no matter the valence, the origin is always assumed to be the patient's personal early childhood experiences transferred into the present moment as part of the therapeutic relationship. In this early model of psychoanalysis, the doctor/analyst was assumed to be neutral, open, and curious about the patient who brings his or her emotional issues for treatment. Whatever happens during the therapeutic hour stems directly from the patient. For example, when I greet a patient at our first meeting, I would assume, from a classically psychoanalytic point of view, that their demeanor is caused by their inner world and personal history not my greeting. This may be a mistaken assumption, which we will explore in the more relational world of Chapter 7.

Frame

The "frame" is another aspect of the early therapy model, and it continues to this day, in some form, between every therapist and client. The frame is a combination of the agreements between the clinician and the patient and the boundaries imposed by the analyst (Langs, 1978). So, within the traditional frame, you—the client or patient—agree to come at a certain time on certain days of the week. You own that time and pay for it, whether you use it or not. What you pay and when you pay also is an agreement. Among the rules imposed by the analyst is that there will be no contact outside of the frame, as that would contaminate the transference. Any change of an appointment or discussion about fee needs to be handled within the time you have together so it can be analyzed and understood. For example, you might think that you won't come to your session tomorrow because it is your spouse's birthday. Then, in the course of the discussion, you might discover that you were disappointed in yesterday's analytic conversation and would prefer not to come another time this week and risk further disappointment. Having reflected more deeply on the situation, your choice to not come is more nuanced. Yes, it is your spouse's birthday and, yes, you don't want to feel disappointment. This is how a good analysis can help each of us understand ourselves more fully. Such complexity of insight into ourselves is one of the overarching gifts that Freud gave us.

Furthering this mode of nuanced thinking, Freud proposed the notion of "negation," where the patient often means the opposite of what he or she is saying (Freud, 1925). "I love my mother and had a wonderful childhood," is an overly simplistic example of defenses keeping the patient from the truth of the instinctual drives, which push for wanting and hating and not getting and guilt about both hating and loving and a whole host of complex feelings masked by the simple sentence above. In Freud's vision, these fundamental instinctual drives were too harsh to bear and had to be denied and hidden. Classically, the analyst needs to hold the attitude that the patient does not speak the full truth about himself or his situation (Orange, 2011). The analyst is deeply attuned, attending to every utterance, open to excavating each story in search of the "deeper truth."

Classical analysis also eschewed any form of physical contact whatsoever between patient and analyst. For some analysts, even a handshake would be too gratifying or supportive and would undermine the task of confronting yourself and understanding the depth of your own needs and impulses. In an effort to stay neutral, to become the reflecting mirror, the analyst refrained from offering any personal information to the patient.

Freud became convinced that people were not what they presented themselves to be. The good, upstanding, competent householder had dark and hidden aspects that he did not show to others and likely did not recognize as a part of himself. Freud came to believe that we are full of secrets and conflicts—not just secrets from others, but secrets from ourselves, and not just conflicts with others, but conflicts within. Moreover, many of these secrets and conflicts were unconscious. He believed that he knew his patients—even on first meeting—better than they knew themselves. He knew that they had sexual needs and aggressive impulses, and that they were likely guilty about both. He knew they carried dissociated memories and were likely troubled by compelling fantasies. It was his commitment to uncover these hidden aspects that formed the therapeutic bond and the process of uncovering these heretofore unknown aspects that would allow the patient to become more balanced and integrated. At least, that was the theory (Orange, 2011).

Repetition compulsion

Another gift Freud gave us is the notion of the "repetition compulsion" (Freud, 1914). He found that when his patients failed to consciously remember what they had repressed, they would unconsciously enact and re-enact their history. This repetition is far more than recreating the familiar.

Jess enacts her anxiety through her chronically tentative stance in my office. She is unconsciously repeating her earlier experiences in a present context. Freud suggests that, in neurosis, the repetition compulsion can override the pleasure principle, creating misery and pain instead. Initially, he believed that the intent of a repetition compulsion was to restore an earlier way of being in the world, recreating the familiar. It is as if I try to get my needs met by insistently making the same demand over and over. In Jess' case, she is transmitting, "Reassure me, make me safe," without any conscious awareness that she is unsafe in certain contexts. Freud later proposed that this repetition might be a part of mastery—that is, learning to be active rather than passive in an upsetting and disturbing situation. A further suggestion was that the repetition compulsion represents an incapacity to learn due to a traumatic event. No doubt, there is truth in all of these scenarios. Our very human behavior of recreating relationships and events that do not satisfy continues to bring people into therapy, and, sadly, these patterns are often very difficult to shift. Freud's powers of observations were remarkably astute, even though, today, we have a different understanding of what is driving the process.

Classic technique

Throughout the years, as Freud listened to his patients and theorized—arguably privileging theory over listening—he created what became known as the classic psychoanalytic technique (Greenson, 1967). Patients were instructed to lay on a couch while he sat out of sight, listening carefully. His instructions were to talk about anything that came to mind and then to free associate to the thoughts that emerged. Freud believed that his "neutrality" and the non-directedness of this method would ensure that what occurred during the session would reveal the patient's personal conflicts while allowing him, Freud, to stay autonomous. This combination, Freud believed, would be the most direct route to the source of trouble. His intent when speaking was to offer an interpretation—usually a connection between the present dilemma and a past conflict—that he felt would be useful. The interpretation would open the door to the unconscious and its conflicts. Additionally, it would ensure the relational needs of the patient were not gratified in any way.

As Freud analyzed his patient's free associations, he discovered both sides of the problem as he envisioned it: the secrets or memories that were the source of the pain and the defenses that were the protection from painful awareness of that same secret or memory. Analysis became the process of focusing on what was happening in the session between doctor and patient, explaining the transference, uncovering the various defenses, and eventually welcoming the private, secret impulses that arise to make themselves known (Storr, 1989).

Jess' struggle involves always being frightened of other people while, at the same time, longing for intimate human connection. The conflict was enacted each time we met: Her negative transference said I hated her, that she must reveal as little as possible, and that she was in danger; while her lived experience with me was that, together, we sought to figure out her past and that, during this hour, I had not harmed her. I would ask that directly at the end of each session: "Did I do or say anything that harmed you or felt 'off' in some way?" For several years, her

(continued)

(continued)

defenses stayed on high alert to protect her from more harm. At the end of each session, she would rise, shake her head, and repeat some version of: "When you get to know me, you, too, will hate me."

My work with Suzi unfolds differently. Her positive transference assumes that I see her as important and worthwhile. Her defenses are designed to deflect any speck of "less than perfect." If I ask her about her impact on the others in her life, including me, she struggles. She maintains a sense of entitlement, wanting to be seen in only a positive light. As a result, other people are rather colorless and two-dimensional. It emerges that, in her inner world, she is in technicolor and everyone else is in black and white. Suzi is convinced that only by staying shiny and positive will she attract friends and a partner, and she deflects any feedback that challenges her very positive self-image.

Classic technique, continued

For many years, Freud's classical technique was the only available form of therapy for problems of the mind or emotions. In its traditional form, patients met with their analysts many times a week. It is hard for anyone who has not experienced this to imagine how healing it can be to have three to five hours each week where you talk to someone who listens intently and is (theoretically) focused only on you. You learn a lot about yourself as you hear yourself talk and begin to notice the reoccurring themes and repeated issues that trouble you the most. With the right analyst, it is a powerful approach to the "examined life"—the life most worth living. Yet, there are times when issues do not resolve themselves, when depression does not lift, nor mourning lighten, nor anxieties calm, when the interpretations offered do not feel accurate or meaningful. Then the analysis is stuck without enough consciousness and integration.

Dreams

While Freud was creating and practicing psychoanalysis, he was conducting his own self-analysis, seeking to discover his own conflicts and challenges. He also was writing prodigiously. Freud wrote long letters, scientific articles, and impressively long and important books. *The Interpretation of Dreams* (1900) remains among his most famous, the first book to become a classic on dreams and their meanings. From his own self-analysis, Freud had noticed that his dreams were important sources of information elucidating his own secret inner workings. For example, in an early dream, he examined a current patient and found that the reason she was not progressing as he had hoped was because another doctor had left a syringe inside her. In the dream, he felt very relieved that it was not his fault; it was someone else's. As he thought about the dream, he realized that it relieved his guilt that he was failing her, that it was a wish-fulfillment story. Based on experiences like this, in his final formulation, dreams, both the night dream and the daydream, were almost always a form of wish fulfillment, either a current wish or an unresolved wish from childhood. (Storr, 1989). This idea became central to therapeutically successful interpretations. Over time, the enormous importance Freud placed on dreams and their interpretations is captured by his famous phrase that they are "the royal road to the unconscious."

For Freud and classical analysts, the dream always exists on two levels. The "manifest content" was the images remembered and reported, and the "latent content" was what the dream was really about, the wishes that it was revealing. In his understanding, dreaming was necessary in order to stay asleep. As a result, the dream translates current issues into various non-threatening images, allowing the dreamer to continue sleeping.

At first, Freud wanted to discover the universal language of the dream world, but he soon relinquished that idea, concluding that dream symbols are more personal than universal. Nevertheless, in his mind, the symbols in dreams tended to point towards sexual and/or aggressive themes, the forces of the id expressing themselves while the ego and superego are at rest.

Developmental model

In additional to a generalized id, Freud hypothesized that children come with drives (Storr, 1989). The first primary drive he referred to as "oral," the need for food to survive. The baby's first sense of life itself is around his/her mouth and the satisfaction that the mouth provides. Hunger brings tension; satiation gives relief.

The second focus of orientation for the child comes into play towards the end of the second year of life: how to manage urination and defecation. For Freud, this was the first big socialization issue, the first power struggle. He called it the "anal drive." This period of life represents several conflicts for the child, both internally and with his caregivers. The child both wants to please and not to please his "important others." He needs to assert his autonomy and to fit into the family. Again, we find the experience of tension, holding in urine and feces and then the experience of relief with evacuation. Gathering the mental and physical self-control to manage these is a major developmental achievement for the child.

The next bodily focus for the child in the Freudian model occurs when the child discovers his genitals and becomes interested in the pleasures to be found there. This is far more obvious in little boys than in little girls, but most children do come to the realization that this is a special part of their body, somewhat different from the rest. The genital drive is a time of integration in this model. The child relinquishes the pleasures of the oral and anal stages of life and begins to develop him- or herself as a sexual being. In Freud's way of thinking, when we are healthy—that is, not neurotic—the new replaces the old; maturity replaces infantile needs and wishes.

Oedipal complex

The "Oedipal conflict" is the apex of Freud's developmental theory, and was, for him, the key to understanding the drives of sexuality and aggression along with the creation of guilt (Mitchell & Black, 1995). Freud believed that around age five or six, the child began to sexually desire the parent of the opposite sex and, as a result of this, the same-sexed parent became a rival. At this time, the male child in particular can come into a terrific conflict involving both strong desire—wanting Mom all to himself—and terrible fear—if Dad finds out, he will retaliate. Freud hypothesized that the Oedipal conflict was resolved through the force of "castration anxiety," pushing the child to realize he must renounce his sexual desires in order to remain whole—literally, bodily—and stay in the family. The gender bias of Freud's time becomes especially apparent here. Obviously, fear of castration is less likely to motivate little girls. Despite these glaring limits and concerns, the idea of the Oedipal complex gives us a first psycho-biological understanding of deep-seated guilt (I want what I can't have and might be punished for even wanting it), so with some patients it still deserves our honest consideration.

No one, including Freud, believes that children actually desire sexual intercourse with their parents. However, it is clear that many children romantically adore their opposite-sex parent at this stage of development. Little girls do fantasize, sometimes quite openly, about "marrying Daddy," and little boys do compete with Dad for Mom's time and affection. I once worked with a family in which the little boy, about age four, clung to his mother every evening when his father came home, saying, "My sweet Mama and you can't have her." This evening ritual went on for about six months before simply disappearing. We know from other perspectives that children have elaborate fantasies involving their "good parent" and their "bad parent," often wanting unlimited time, attention, and affection from the good one. Because of these experiences, I believe that the idea of an Oedipal complex can highlight a developmental issue that could induce unconscious fear and guilt in some adults.

I can look at Suzi through the lens of the Oedipal conflict as the child who "won" the father from the mother. When we met, any guilt she felt for this winning was totally unconscious; she was only proud and pleased at being the favorite. Suzi had little empathy for her siblings or her mother. Her inner world consisted of only her and her father, with no room for others. As we slowly unpacked the consequences of being the favorite, Suzi discovered that when allowing some feelings of guilt to emerge, she came into contact with tender feelings of sadness and empathy. This awakening of her tenderness nourished and improved her connections with others.

Mourning

Freud also started the conversation around mourning (1917a). Mourning has always been considered of great importance in any analysis or depth psychology. What I want to note here is that in his first consideration of the subject, he wrote that mourning (not melancholia) was a healthy, conscious process and could be completed. That is, slowly the mourner would sever ties with whatever he has lost, freeing his energy, his libido, to attach to new others. Undoubtedly, the mourner is changed by the experience of the loss and that transformation is beyond personal control. Many other writers, including Anna Freud, his daughter, have augmented his theory, and I know from personal experience that completion is not really possible with significant losses: mourning comes in waves, often for many years. However, I want to note that, again, Freud took the risk to put ideas into the public sphere for us to consider and discuss.

Later theory

By the 1920s, Freud's map of the human psyche was very complex. He had started with what is called the "topographical model," wherein the "acceptable" senses of self rest on a much larger unconscious and unacceptable sense of self, which included sexual and aggressive impulses, repressed wishes, and unknown memories. Freud next gave us his "structural model." Each of our three inner resources—id, ego, and superego—represents different ways of being and acting in the world. The id contains our bodily excitements, our passions, and our impulses. The ego is our "reality tester." The ego asks, "Can I really have what my 'id' wants?" Our superego represents the set of values we strive to live up to and frequently fail to live up to. In our superego, our goals and aspirations share space with our critical voices and our self-doubts. Freud believed it was possible to transform our primitive drive-based id into our civilized ego. He famously said, "Where id is, ego shall be," and he wanted that possibility for each of his patients. His model was economic; that is, there is only a fixed or set amount of energy moving among the three aspects of psyche.

Freud's developmental model is a meta frame for the unfolding of what has come to be known as the "formative years." In Freud's imagination, the baby is pushed by drives through these early erogenous zones of oral, anal, and phallic. Developmentally, adults could be stuck at any of these levels with too much of their libido, or life energy, bound into neediness, compulsiveness, or the guilt and fear of the triangle of the Oedipal conflict. When libido is stuck and development is arrested, the adult patient is not free to create or choose for himself in the present. Rather, he is stuck in historical or archaic issues, which will be enacted in the transference of the analytic dyad.

Freud initially believed in and hoped for personal transformation for his patients. He began his career as a neurologist at a time when it seemed possible that science was destined to solve all human problems. He also lived in Vienna, Austria, a city that appeared—at least on the surface—to be full of tolerance and diversity. Living through World War I and the rise of Nazism, which forced him to leave Vienna for London at the end of his life, along with the death of his beloved daughter, Sophie, shadowed his initial optimism that human beings can manage id impulses and create a meaningful existence, fulfilling his twin goals of love and work.

Freud was the first speaker in the conversations that form the following chapters. He gives us our first structures of mind. His profound and wide-ranging intellectual legacy explored questions about our basic nature and needs, our motivations, and our conflicts, and sought answers to our emotional suffering and the mechanisms of emotional healing. He impacted far more than the study of the mind and what would become psychotherapy. Until only recently, all of the thinkers presented here, no matter how different their theory, considered themselves to be part of the Freudian lineage.

Today, many of the details of his theory have been discarded; however, the raw framework remains remarkably robust. Modern neuroscience has confirmed that we are born with a very complex brain, unfinished at birth and completed only in the context of the family. Much of the functioning of that brain remains unconscious. At birth, we are a bundle of needs and impulses that must be fulfilled, or we will die. The formative years are crucial to adult well-being. We all get stuck in unhelpful ways. Freud outlined these aspects of human life in broad strokes, initiating both the conversations and the research foundational to modern life.

Key concepts Chapter 1

Castration anxiety – what the little boy fears in the fantasy of excluding his father in order to have an exclusive relationship with his mother

Defenses – the patterns each of us creates in order to avoid psychic pain and vulnerability

Drive-conflict model – according to Freud, sexuality and aggression are basic to instinctual life and they need discharge either in fantasy or literally, creating conflict with others

Ego – in the structural model of id, ego, and superego, the ego is the mediator between the drives of the id and the superego ideals of the family and culture

Ego ideal – a fantasy created by the growing self of how I should be or wish to be; always unrealistic, but important as a human striving

Eros – Freud's term for the positive life force including sexuality and sensuality

Frame – the conscious agreements between analyst/therapist and patient including time and money

Free association – the invitation to speak whatever comes to mind without censoring

Guilt – is explained by both the Oedipal theory and the gaps between the superego ideals and the ego's ability to live up to those ideals

Hysteria – historically referred to a collection of vague, unaccountable symptoms, such as excessive emotionality, attention-seeking behavior, and bouts of amnesia, found exclusively in women

Id – in the structural model of id, ego, and superego, the id is the basic driver of unconscious, instinctual life

Latent content – what the dream is pointing to after being understood in a deeper, richer way using both free associations and interpretations

Libido – the energy of Eros and sexuality; positive life force or energy

Manifest content – the images and narrative remembered from a dream

Mourning – the process of grieving and integrating a loss into one's psychic structure

Negation – saying the opposite of what is true; a Freudian defense

Negative transference – experiencing the analyst/therapist in an automatically negative light

Oedipal complex – a developmental stage wherein the young child desires an exclusive relationship with the parent of the opposite sex and fears retribution from the parent of the same sex

Positive transference – experiencing the analyst/therapist in an automatically positive, even idealized, light

Repetition compulsion – our capacity to endlessly repeat a traumatic or distressing pattern over and over in dreams and/or behavior

Repression – one of Freud's basic defenses: our human capacity to put painful emotions or experiences out of awareness

Structural model – the interplay of the id, ego, and superego—psychic structures hypothesized by Freud to explain what he was experiencing as an analyst

Superego – in the structural model of id, ego, and superego, the superego holds the ideals and the injunctions from parents and culture

Thanatos – the death instinct including our self-destructive tendencies

Topographical model – the idea that the conscious is but a small part of our psychic structure and the unconscious is much larger and more in control than we imagine

Transference – Freud noticed and named the fact that our first experiences as infants unconsciously shape how we relate to others in the future, especially important others or figures in authority

Wish fulfillment – originally the idea that a dream was pointing to what the dreamer truly wanted

References

Bloom, H. (1986) Freud, the greatest modern writer. *New York Times Book Review*, March 23, pp. 1, 26–27.

Brenner, C. (1955, 1974) *An Elementary Textbook of Psychoanalysis*. Garden City, NY: Anchor Press/Doubleday.

Einstein, A., Nathan, O., & Norden, H. (1960) *Einstein on Peace*. New York: Simon & Schuster.

Freud, A. (1935) *Psychoanalysis for Teachers and Parents*. Boston: Beacon Press.

Freud, S. (1896) The aetiology of hysteria. *Standard Edition*, vol. 3. London: Hogarth.

Freud, S. (1900) *The Interpretation of Dreams*. *Standard Edition*, vols 4–5. London: Hogarth.

Freud, S. (1901, 1990) *The Psychopathology of Everyday Life*. New York: Norton.

Freud, S. (1905) *Three Essays on the Theory of Sexuality*. *Standard Edition*, vol. 7. London: Hogarth.

Freud, S. (1912) The dynamics of transference. *Standard Edition*, vol. 12 London: Hogarth.

Freud, S. (1914) Remembering, repeating and working through. *Standard Edition*, vol. 12. London: Hogarth.

Freud, S. (1917a) Mourning and melancholia. *Standard Edition*, vol. 14. London: Hogarth.

Freud, S. (1917b) *Introductory Lectures on Psychoanalysis*. *Standard Edition*, vols 15–16. London: Hogarth.

Freud, S. (1920) *Beyond the Pleasure Principle*. *Standard Edition*, vol. 18. London: Hogarth.

Freud, S. (1925) Negation. *International Journal of Psychoanalysis*, 6, 235–239.

Greenson, R.R. (1967) *The Technique and Practice of Psychoanalysis*, vol. 1. New York: International Universities Press.

Herman, J. (1992) *Trauma and Recovery*. New York: Basic Books.

Langs, R. (1978) *The Listening Project*. New York: Aronson.

Mitchell, S. & Black, M. (1995) *Freud and Beyond*, New York: Basic Books.

Orange, D. (2011) *The Suffering Stranger*. New York: Routledge.

Storr, A. (1989) *Freud: A Very Short Introduction*. Oxford: Oxford University Press.

2

THE BRIDGE BETWEEN FREUD AND MODERN PSYCHOANALYSIS

Freud desired to leave a clear legacy. He wanted to appoint a successor and have that individual continue his work true to his intent. Along the way, he appointed and discarded several possibilities, including Carl Jung (1875–1961) and Sándor Ferenczi (1873–1933), both of whom are important in their own right but not part of my so-called family tree. Freud never did achieve his desire. There is no clear legacy, no one true Freudian school of thought although some analysts still hue closely to the original model. Therefore, I have divided his legacy into the six schools that are active in the world of English-speaking psychoanalysis today, all of which continue the conversations he started, albeit in very different ways.

Because of World War II, Freud and most of his followers had to leave continental Europe, and many found their way to London. Accordingly, at that time, London became the center of orthodox psychoanalysis, and many of the men and women I will talk about lived there, including Anna Freud, Melanie Klein, Donald "D.W." Winnicott, and John Bowlby.

Freud, Jung, and Ferenczi in Vienna

Freud invited physicians to join his Psychoanalytic Institute in Vienna, Austria, to share his excitement and knowledge about the inner workings of the mind. Both Carl Jung and Sándor Ferenczi were a part of that circle for a time and both left and, in due course, formed their own schools of thought. Both also rejected the Freudian drive theory but for very different reasons. Jung held a less biological, more spiritual view of man. He believed that humans are based in a transpersonal organizing self that guides each of us on a personal journey of

(continued)

(continued)

individuation. His school continues to this day in both Europe and the United States. Very differently, Ferenczi stayed with Freud's original thought that sexual trauma was real and causative in psychological disorders. To Freud's dismay, Ferenczi advocated an active, interpersonal form of psychoanalysis, totally different from Freud's studied neutrality. For many years, he was completely ostracized and discarded from all psychoanalytic thinking. However, today, he is claimed as an important precursor in both theory and practice, especially in the American relational school of thought, and his reputation and importance are now acknowledged (Mitchell & Black, 1995).

It would be logical for Freud's daughter, Anna Freud, to be his heir apparent. After all, he had analyzed her (unthinkable in today's world), she was a well-regarded analyst, and she alone was allowed to take care of him in his dying months in London. However, when she and her father arrived in London just before World War II began, they found a strong and lively psychoanalytic tradition already thriving. Anna, like Melanie Klein, worked in an analytic frame with young children using both words and actions (play houses, drawing, sand trays, and toys) to determine and interpret what was stalling her young patients' development. Even so, Anna and Melanie were always more competitive than collaborative. Anna's school of thought, called ego psychology, continues to be an important force in modern thinking. After the war, she traveled often to the United States and became a powerful influence there (Young-Bruehl, 1988).

Melanie Klein had migrated from Berlin to London in 1926 at the age of 44. She was one of the most brilliant, outspoken, and powerful analysts in London. Although without formal education, she bore an impressive psychoanalytic pedigree, having been analyzed by two famous analysts, Ferenczi during World War I and later by Karl Abraham. She and others formulated the basics of what is now called object-relations theory, moving Freud's developmental focus back in time from the Oedipal triangle to babyhood issues. The object-relations focus is not on guilt but rather on problems of fragmentation of self. These are now appropriately referred to as pre-Oedipal issues. Freud knew that his techniques were not suitable for people with these early traumas, as they lacked the ego strength to bear the confrontations with the drives. Klein disagreed and created a way to analyze both children and adults suffering from these very early issues (Grosskurth, 1986).

The third British school I will discuss centers on Donald Winnicott, who also was analyzed by two influential analysts: first by James Strachey in the 1920s and then by Joan Riviere in the late 1930s (Rodman, 2003). He is considered to be part of Klein's object-relations school of thought and, indeed, he was embedded in that model for his early professional life. However, his evolving contributions are so strikingly different that, to my mind, he and his associates form a third distinctive line from Freud. During World War II, the British psychoanalytic school splintered, with Kleinians forming one branch and the Anna Freudians forming another branch. Winnicott, among others, Michael Balint, Ronald Fairbairn, and Harry Guntrip, created the middle or independent group, the third branch. This arrangement continues to this day.

Even though he was trained as a psychoanalyst around the same time, John Bowlby's calling was to study children and their primary needs, a theoretical position that he called attachment theory. Using a research style that is close to ethnology, he theorized that children need close contact with a primary other in order to fully develop. Thus, his focus was on the observable, real relationship between parents and children, rather than the inner struggles and conflicts first outlined by Freud. His insistence on the concrete, real relationship ostracized him from the prevailing analytic communities post-World War II and for many decades thereafter (Fonagy, 2001). Currently, his attachment theory is considered a key to psychological healing within most analytic traditions. In my lineage model, Bowlby forms the sixth branch.

American psychoanalysis has a complex history all its own. I am interested in two branches that are thriving today: psychology of the self, the work of Kohut, and relational psychoanalysis, the lineage of Sullivan. All of the English traditions, as well as "classical" analysis, the truest to the original Freudian model and intent, exist in the United States, but these two strictly American schools have had the most powerful influence on psychoanalysis and psychotherapy in this country and certainly on my thinking and clinical style.

Like Freud, Kohut fled Vienna in 1939. After finishing medical school and analysis in Chicago, he became a traditional analyst. By the 1950s, his focus had become empathy, empathic immersion, developmental deficits, and narcissism. He modified the conventional technique to suit his new emphasis, which produced a very different stance from Freud's total neutrality (Strozier, 2001). His lineage is the fourth branch of my tree.

Sullivan—my fifth branch—was the other American who dramatically changed psychoanalysis and psychotherapy. Sullivan called himself a neo-Freudian, but his work would not be recognized by a traditional analyst, either in theory or in practice. Ultimately, Sullivan's theory was neither biological nor drive-based. He focused on the interpersonal world in which people live. In his view, we are always in a context and always needing to find a way to ward off anxiety. Sullivan and his followers saw therapy as a relationship, not an authority figure treating a patient (Perry, 1982).

The rest of this book will be devoted to my understanding of these six branches of Freud's lineage and how they impact current thinking, as well as their current interrelationships with both mindfulness and neuroscience. This is a selective, though representational, list of contributors whose ideas have most helped and influenced my clinical work. Each contributor offered more ideas than I detail, and each branch has many more contributors than I mention. This is both a personally chosen lineage and, at the same time, an accurate history of developments in the world of psychoanalysis.

Two further notes:

Until the 1950s in Europe, becoming an analyst was contingent only on being analyzed yourself. This was the apprentice model, and many of the people discussed here were trained in this way. At some point, most who wanted to declare themselves practicing analysts were further required to present a paper to the society of their home city. In places without such a society, individuals would have an analysis and simply begin to use the theory and technique in their own way. There were no required educational standards in Europe. However, for several decades in America, a doctor of medicine degree, or MD, was a prerequisite to becoming a practicing analyst, forcing psychoanalysis into the field of psychiatry. Later, in both America and Europe, training institutes were created, some requiring a related training in medicine, social work, or psychology, all requiring a formal analysis, clinical supervision, and course work beginning by reading Freud.

Wherever it is relevant, I have mentioned participation in either or both of the Great Wars, as I believe such a traumatic experience profoundly influences the human psyche. Many of the men who later became analysts served in the military. To see combat changes a person forever. Moreover, a disproportionate number of early psychoanalysts were of Jewish origin, including Freud himself. The focus in the second war to eliminate their entire race had to have had a great impact on their thinking about human nature. These events were part of Freud's life, and his book, *Civilization and Its Discontents*, bears witness to his struggle to account for their horrific impact.

Key concepts Chapter 2

Attachment theory – Bowlby's assertion that the infant needs consistent care in order to develop physically and psychologically

Developmental deficits – the consequence of stalled development due to poor care in early childhood resulting in missing resiliency or ego strength

Ego psychology – one of the branches to evolve which privileges the ego and ego strength over the more primitive drives of the original Freudian theory

Ego strength – the capacity of the ego or self (depending on the psychoanalytic school) to manage both inner impulses and needs as well as outer stressors

Empathic immersion – the technique or style developed by Kohut to deeply connect with the suffering of others

Empathy – our inbuilt capacity to emotionally understand others and therefore to connect with them. An important term in the lexicon of self psychology

Middle or independent school – the group of analysts who did not side with either Anna Freud or Melanie Klein, who insisted that the infant was object-seeking, not drive discharge-seeking and that the relationship with the analyst needed to involve care

Narcissism – a term used to describe a continuum of characteristics from healthy agency to pathological self-centeredness

Neo-Freudian – schools of thought that have derived from Freud, but modified both theory and technique

Object-relations theory – an in-depth understanding of mental life as based on the infant's first experiences with others, specifically family

Pre-Oedipal issues – inner dynamics of mental life formed in the first five years of life.

Relational psychoanalysis – the analytic school evolving from the work of Sullivan that emphasizes the importance of both real and imagined relationships from the beginning of life as the cause of emotional pathology

Self psychology – the analytic school of Kohut, noting that the struggle to be valued emotionally and understood first by family, then by others, creates meaning and growth throughout life

References

Fonagy, P. (2001) *Attachment Theory and Psychoanalysis*. New York: Other Press.

Grosskurth, P. (1986). *Melanie Klein: Her World and Her Work*. New York: Knopf.

Mitchell, S. & Black, M. (1995) *Freud and Beyond*, New York: Basic Books.

Perry, H.S. (1982) *Psychiatrist of America: The Life of Harry Stack Sullivan*. Cambridge, MA: Harvard University Press.

Rodman, F.R. (2003) *Winnicott: Life and Work*. Cambridge, MA: Perseus.

Strozier, C.B. (2001) *Heinz Kohut: The Making of a Psychoanalyst*. New York: Farrar, Straus & Giroux.

Young-Bruehl, E. (1988) *Anna Freud: A Biography*. New York: Norton.

3

MELANIE KLEIN

Life is terrifying, and we must survive

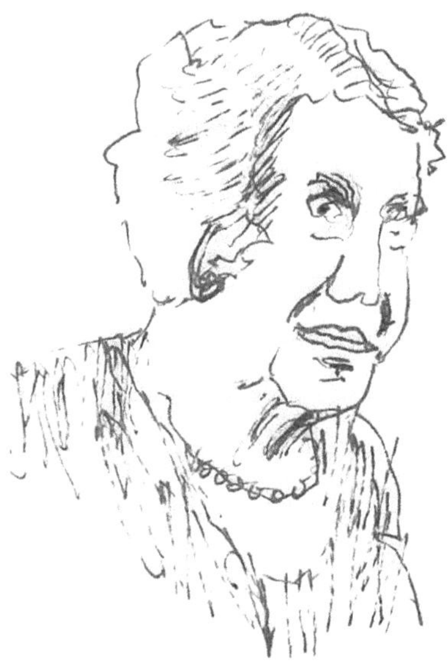

Melanie Klein

Melanie Klein (1882–1960) had arrived in London from Berlin in 1926 long before Freud and Anna were forced to move there. In addition to fleeing anti-Semitism, she was unhappily married, separated, and had three children to support. She was working with children through play therapy and devising her own theories about children, play, and the unconscious. She quickly became a leading figure in the British psychoanalytic community. Klein considered herself a true Freudian and insisted that her work was an elaboration and extension of his. However, for her the Freudian drives had an object (most often the breast or the mother) and not only the pleasure of discharge. Additionally, she theorized about what she called part-objects, as the infant's mind in the first years of life was not developed enough to realize more than the function he needed (Grosskurth, 1986). Although she used the language of drive theory and other Freudian concepts, her writings and practice took her in a distinctly different, and, developmentally, much earlier, direction. Over time, she decided that her concept of the depressive position beginning later in the first year of life is the nodal point for further development, not the Oedipal period of ages five or six (Mitchell & Black, 1995).

Freud was concerned with elaborating and understanding the structures of the mind as the child moved through developmental stages—oral, anal, phallic—culminating in the Oedipal triangle, which was the focus of his therapeutic work. In dramatic contrast, Klein was preoccupied with the primitive agonies, the life and death dramas of babyhood, and how these related to the psychological struggles of adults (Segal, 1979). She always worked with children, and she, like Freud, analyzed her own children, using her work with her youngest in a thinly disguised form as her paper for admission to the Budapest Society (Grosskurth, 1986). While shocking to our current mindset, this was not remarkable at the time.

By focusing on children, Klein moved both the practice and the working metaphor from the guilty six-year-old engaged with incestuous and aggressive impulses to that of the infant struggling to survive while at the mercy of another (Klein & Riviere, 1964). Her ideas had a huge impact in the London community. In shifting the focus to the first years of life, Klein believed that psychoanalysis could help a much different level of suffering. Freud had acknowledged that his way of working was not suitable for these very early pre-Oedipal issues, as the sufferer did not have enough ego strength to bear looking at the pain without getting lost in it. Klein insisted this was possible and, in fact, for her, the true focus of the analytic project (Mitchell & Black, 1995).

A reminder on Freudian drive theory

At its most fundamental, Freud's drive theory is simple, mechanistic, and hydraulic. According to this theory, human psychic energy is generated by the libido or biological life force and channeled into drives by instinctual needs. A drive has both a biological and a psychological component. Tension is created when the need is not satisfied. The drive needs to discharge its tension—that is the pleasure. Freud was intellectually interested in the big dichotomy of Eros and Thanatos, not the more physiological drives of bodily life (Brenner, 1955, 1974).

A changing analytic culture

Early psychoanalysis had very different boundaries and mores from what we would accept today. For example, the masculine was the standard and assumed superior; friends would analyze each other or each other's children. Guntrip talked often with Fairbairn, his first analyst, about his ongoing analysis with Winnicott. All of this was part of the analytic culture of the time.

Like Freud, Klein's theories evolved over decades, and she seems to have had little interest in reconciling various formulations. Of course, her theories were influenced by her own life events, especially the very difficult ones: abandonment by her husband, the death of a son, the estrangement of her eldest daughter in the analytic wars, and her own frequent depressions (Grosskurth, 1986). I believe these traumatic losses encouraged her to understand the horrific pain of the negative emotional defenses to terrible loss and the need to develop gratitude and reparation.

She believed in an a priori inner world populated by what might be called "memory traces" and phantasies of bodies and body parts. She wrote that the infant has instinctual knowledge about the existence of his mother and is primed to be in relationship with his mother (Klein & Riviere, 1964). Among her most important contributions is her conceptualization of the infant's built-in drive to both incorporate and to expel "good" and "bad" objects. In this context, the word "object" refers to someone or something that has significance to the baby's emerging sense of self and is carried within the baby's imagination (Klein, J., 1987). Objects are structures that endure and are active in the child's inner world. They are initially rudimentary and primitive. A newborn is only equipped to experience its most basic needs. It is preoccupied with survival, which means getting food and being held, warmed, and protected. An infant neither knows nor cares that another person performs these functions. The baby cares only that the functions happen and at the right time, which is *when needed in this moment*. Klein hypothesized that a baby responds to "part-objects"—these are typically body parts or their substitutes, which young children experience as meeting their basic needs (Klein, J., 1987). The breast or the bottle is such a part object because it exists to gratify immediate need. This process of gratification creates the tie between what is to become the "self" of the baby and the "other" or object.

Bad objects

Objects are experienced as "bad" if they are not present when needed or, in some way, cause pain. The Kleinian stance is that the infant is forced to think about and actively deal with frustrations before pleasurable experiences; therefore, bad objects are internally conceptualized first. Pleasurable experiences continue the initial baby–mother merger. Thus, frustration prompts the individuation process. Like Freud, Klein believed that the tiny baby experienced himself as merged with whoever took care of him. To grow a "self" is to individuate, to become your own person. By experiencing the "rupture" provided by a bad experience, the infant starts to relinquish that merger in favor of a more separate stance. Therefore, some experience with "bad objects" is key to growth and individuation, too much is overwhelming and forces the infant away from his true unfolding (Mitchell & Black, 1995).

Klein maintained that the infant lives in a split world of the good and the bad. In this primitive mode of "thinking," when the world is good, all is good. I am good; the source of the food is good; Mommy is good. The opposite also is true: When the baby is uncomfortable: everything is bad—the baby itself, the source of food, everything. There is no time and no memory of things being different. What is just is and always has been. Klein astutely realized that, at the beginning of life, this way of being in the world is normal: Either everything is utterly OK, or it is terribly not OK. If development does not go well enough, adults will often continue to "split" events and objects into stark categories, such as when we idealize and then devalue people and things (Mitchell & Black, 1995).

For Klein, the infant is creating "phantasies" from birth on (Segal, 1979). She observed that tiny babies do not differentiate between reality and imagination. She theorized that the infant is creating phantasies in order to ward off terror—the intense anxiety that she posited threatens the baby's survival and that, for her, is always the infant's first experience of life. If the baby does not get enough human contact or enough food, it "knows" it will die. So, these terrors are biologically built in and, in a way, ensure these basic needs are met.

Klein did not view these phantasies as based on interactions with the real (m)other. Like her mentor Freud, she viewed all ideation at this stage of life as based only on internal life. She was clear that there were many inner objects and many inner object relationships, but they were all an inherent part of a priori knowledge.

A jump into the future

Klein's contention that such black and white extremes are all an infant's physiology can manage is one way of looking at the data provided by current neuroscience. This body of work will be discussed in detail later in this book. It shows us that the first year of life is dominated by the primitive hind- and limbic brain, where experiences and impulses are immediate, total, and timeless (Siegel, 2007). When life is dominated by this most primitive part of our complex brain, it is analogous to Klein's primitive agonies and the realm of phantasy.

Phantasy and fantasy

For Klein, phantasy is the baby's state of mind at the beginning of life when it cannot distinguish between its inner world of imagination and outer reality. Phantasies come from inner drives and instincts (Segal, 1979). In contrast, a fantasy is a reverie or daydream that we all create, often about an imagined future or re-doing an unpleasant event. This type of fantasy may include elements of phantasy living and thinking. Some writers do not make this distinction.

Freud was working with and discussing a more mature psyche, one with discrete impulses and objects. Klein saw that for tiny, vulnerable, dependent babies, libidinal and aggressive impulses are entire ways of experiencing oneself as good, loved, and loving or as bad, hated, and destructive. Kleinian theory is addressing the subjective sense that the infant experiences itself as able to create and destroy this split world, making the world of the good and the bad through its aggressive impulses, which for her dominate this time of life. The infant has neither a fully developed psyche nor brain; rather, it lives through its raw biological impulses. In her understanding, this is not a developmental stage to be outgrown, but a "position" that is the template and foundation for much of life (Mitchell & Black, 1995).

This is another marked difference from Freud. He conceived of a developmental sequence where, at least ideally, primitive structures and ideation are transcended and replaced by more advanced and rational ways of thinking. Adults could manifest primitive aspects, but to Freud's mind, these are explained by a "fixation" of libido (life energy) at that stage. Freud required at least the capacity for rational thought for his process to work.

Kleinian positions

Klein posited that our minds are always in one of two positions, both of which manifest at the beginning of life and remain available throughout life (Grosskurth, 1986). She named the first, the paranoid-schizoid position. This platform is a universal part of all of us and is the source of our primitive emotions and defenses. It is the part of us that blames, hates, and is capable of scapegoating. From this position, we will fight to overcome a perceived threat, or we will take "flight," to get away from a sensed danger. From this position, the world is very unsafe (Mitchell & Black, 1995).

As I understand it, this first primitive state of being does not differentiate whether sensation is coming from inside the body or outside, or whether the received information is a current perception or a memory. Whether child or adult, a person in the paranoid-schizoid position finds that life lacks continuity. There is no flow of time—no past and future. The impact or force of the present controls and darkens both the past and the future. Imagine the intensity of a gas pain in your gut. As adults, we know what it is, that it is inside of us and that most likely it will go away. Thanks to our developing brain and lived experience, we grow perspective and the ability to tolerate and wait. The tiny baby does not have such possibilities. It has only intense pain. For the tiny baby, the pain has always been there and will never go away. It is timeless in a very negative way. When an "outside force" changes the baby's position, touches her, does something, then relief comes. This experience, over time, creates a good maternal object, providing what the infant does not have. It takes many experiences of being held and taken care of to learn that such a pain is not life and death, but rather it is a state of being that will change again. However, sometimes no one comes and sometimes nothing helps, leaving the infant in the rage and terror of her split, binary world.

When an adult re-enters this position or way of being (which is always available to us), the universe again splits into "bad" and "good," and the sufferer feels either endangered or enraged. From this position, other people are seen as functions or forces that will either take care of me (good) or harm me (bad). The developmental capacity to experience others as real and separate three-dimensional subjects with a life of their own is not available when we are operating out of the paranoid-schizoid modality (Mitchell & Black, 1995).

Jess has easy access to Klein's paranoid-schizoid state of mind. When she is frightened of upsetting anyone, by having a different opinion or wanting to do a different thing, she physiologically drops into either terror or rage. Jess regularly falls into a panic in my office while knowing rationally that this reaction is not really warranted. The reaction is clearly uncontrollable. Her entire physiology is inflamed. For Jess, to have her own opinion is to be separate, and to be separate when your psyche is struggling with the paranoid-schizoid state of mind is to be abandoned and, therefore, to die. Alternately, having a different opinion can induce her into intense hatred for the other person. Either way, she is alone, left out to die.

Klein also proposed a second, more positive integrating tendency, the depressive position. In her observation, this possibility emerges at around three months of age. Here, we find a pushing for wholeness and the capacity to love, where we are sometimes good, sometimes bad. She noted that an infant is capable of rageful destruction followed by remorse, and then the capacity to repair and to feel gratitude. From this position, she proposed, come the roots of guilt, regret, empathy, and the capacity to mourn—all essential aspects of being a full, complex human being and available much earlier than in the Freudian model (Segal, 1979). This is her depressive position.

She suggests that we move constantly between these two positions. We can always hate the ones we love. We are always in process, always internally fluid. Nothing inside us is a fixed entity or solid. The depressive position in no way indicates depression in the sense of a low mood. Rather, it is a subdued and realistic, yet hopeful state, where miracles are unlikely to happen, and the hard work of integration is lifelong (Klein & Riviere, 1964).

In Klein's world, both of these positions are available from the first year of life forward, and we are in a dialectic with both throughout our lives. As the infant grows into childhood and begins to focus on real others, the psyche learns to hold more and more space for the depressive position. This developmental advance allows repair, mourning, and the possibility of symbolic thinking. For the young child, this development opens the wider world of play and imagination. Stones become play food. The child can be the parent to the doll. From the capacities of the depressive position, self-awareness and thinking about others evolve and consciousness increases. This is both our natural unfolding and what her form of psychoanalysis focuses on re-starting.

When the child cannot complete the developmental task of fully attaining the depressive position, the baby experiences more rage and despair than repair. As a result, there is less overall integration. In these circumstances, the paranoid-schizoid position and the capacity to split the world predominate psychic life. An adult with such a compromised inner world may suffer chaos and desolation in an ongoing cycle throughout life.

Manic defense

Klein has given us many helpful clinical theories. Among the most useful to me is the idea of the manic defense (Mitchell & Black, 1995). In this scenario, the infant has not been helped enough to tolerate these very early feelings of depression following real remorse and regret, Klein's reparation. Remember reparation is designed to restore the connection and the love to the other by experiencing the anxiety and guilt of having harmed that same loved other. By denying the pain of anxiety and guilt, by staying on top of them, the baby, or the adult using this defense, keeps her inner life undisturbed and overly simplified. By being unhelped to experience this deeper emotional pain, the baby and later adult foreclose aspects of her own subjectivity and, very importantly, do not develop fully the empathy necessary to grant others their separate subjectivity. This means that others are not separate and unique people; rather, they are closer to functions, objects that either satisfy or fail current needs. "If this object does not meet my need, the next one will." For someone stuck in this level of development and tied to the manic defense, people are replaceable, whether an assistant or a spouse.

When things don't unfold as she has wished they would, Suzi uses the defense of a manic flight—fleeing from painful feelings, fleeing from envy, fleeing from the despair that she will never have what she really wants. When a project at work misfires, she finds it difficult to talk about what went wrong, what she could do differently, and what she might learn from the mishap. Instead, she jumps to the next good idea or possibility. Sitting with Suzi when she is in this mode is tiring. She talks very fast, refuses to dialogue, and experiences any question as an irritating interruption. Her theme becomes, "The past is the past, there is no point in discussing it; rather, let's move on to the future."

Negative emotions

Klein had a lot to say about our most difficult negative feelings; hate, envy, and greed were her specialties. Klein saw envy as a sadistic expression of destructive impulses, operative from the beginning of life (Klein, 1957; Klein & Riviere, 1964). She believed it had to have a constitutional basis, and, to her mind, some of us are born with too much aggression. As a consequence, for some, envy plays a powerful role in inner life and, therefore, in relational life. In her definition, envy is the fury that another person possesses and enjoys something I want and do not have and believe will never have. Its first object is the breast, and it is the baby's response to frustration. To me, envy means no hope, a very difficult state of being. When in the grip of envy, the individual needs to get it, to take it away from whoever has it in order to survive at least in the psychic sense. If they can't get it, they would prefer to spoil it rather than let the other have it. "*If I can't get it, be more whole, then I certainly don't want you to have it, to have more than me. If I spoil it, at least you are damaged like me.*"

Kleinian envy is a uniquely destructive force with sad and complex byproducts. I want to emphasize that it is strongly linked with an absence of hope. Other emotional companions to envy are humiliation—among the most painful of emotions—and grief. Paradoxically, envy is about wanting the "good" and not being able to have it.

Here is an example of everyday envy that I have witnessed: I am standing in my local supermarket parking lot, admiring a very fancy car. The owner of the car approaches his clearly beloved possession and is about to get in when a man stops, seemingly to admire the car. The two talk for a few minutes and then, as the owner turns to leave, the other man remarks, "I think I read that this model is not considered very safe over 60 miles per hour. Do you find that to be true?" In my imagination, this exchange demonstrates Kleinian envy. It represents an envious attempt to "spoil" the pleasure of the car owner by "damaging" his view of his prized possession. I can easily imagine that the "spoiler" does not and perhaps cannot own such a car. Unconsciously, he wants to damage the unattainable good that the car represents to him.

Envy is about wanting but not being able to possess the good, as it implies no hope of that; envy must spoil the good in order to have some agency, some efficacy. Klein considered it the most destructive of all the primitive impulses, for it destroys all good, including foreclosing unknown possibilities, and harming the sense of a future (Klein, 1957; Mitchell & Black, 1995). When I am working with very destructive or self-destructive people, I usually find a layer of envy, a form of aggression protecting vulnerable self-esteem from further harm and depletion.

Klein usefully contrasts envy, including its lack of hope, to jealousy, where hope is possible (Segal, 1979). When an individual is jealous, they want what the other has, and think it is possible to obtain what the other has. Therefore, hope exists. To be jealous of your shoes, your job, or your marriage, can be part of the motivation to work for another personal version of those shoes, that job, a good marriage.

Consider another client "Mary," whose son is autistic. Mary envies parents who have non-autistic children and, additionally, hates herself for envying them. But, by her report, she "can't help it." Over the past 10 years, Mary has destroyed her social connections by making critical comments about her friends' children. Mary addictively attends to her judgmental and envious inner dialogue regarding the parents in her social circle. She makes no attempt to discriminate or moderate

(continued)

(continued)

her destructive thoughts. She furiously contends that these parents have no right to complain about anything whatsoever. At the same time, she is certain they are not doing a good job in raising their children. Eventually, something of this inner diatribe slips into a conversation and, as a result, her social relationships have eroded.

Mary and her husband are now isolated and unhappy. She wants to extract from her husband all the love and approval she will not give herself and no longer receives from her friends, increasing her aloneness. She is in psychotherapy for the first time. Fortunately, Mary has insight that her words are pushing both her husband and friends away, and she is aware of both her envy and her verbal aggressiveness. As yet, she has no capacity to manage these impulses. My therapeutic task is to give her breathing room around this life-limiting envy, and then gently reveal the lack of hope, deep grief, and painful humiliation that it covers. My goal is to help her realize that she is not a bad person for wishing that she had a different child. Even hating and wanting to destroy the goodness in other families is normal, human, and understandable. I want to widen Mary's focus beyond her toxic envy of other families.

By hypothesizing that all children have hate, envy, and other destructive impulses, Klein helps us normalize these destructive tendencies. Mary needs a lot of support to hold on to a good self with bad actions. When she achieves a tiny triumph of forgiving her negative impulses in a single instance and softening her self-hate, she creates possibility.

Another valuable Kleinian concept is greed. For Klein, greed is an impetuous and insatiable craving, exceeding what the subject needs and what the object is able and willing to give. Its aim is destructive introjection, and individuals held in its thrall can become ruthless in acquisitiveness (Segal, 1979).

"Charlie" exhibits some of what could be called Kleinian greed. Charlie begins every session with a quick addition of his net worth (in the millions) and a weekly story of high-profile purchases. One of anything is never enough. To not have something that he wants is the same as not being good enough, to live in primal shame. So, Charlie needs multiples to feel he is getting the best deal or doing better than someone else. For example, he is very proud of the fact that his six-year-old daughter has over 300 stuffed animals. His little girl having things in excess proves he is "good," both internally and, he hopes, in his mother's and daughter's eyes. Charlie complains that his wife considers him excessively demanding, while he feels his expectations are perfectly reasonable. They clash around his demands on a regular basis. He hates to get up in the morning, and he must face that struggle every workday. His wife rises first to organize the kids for school, and he finds

it reasonable for her to open the curtains and bring him a coffee to help him get started. Her position is she has children to take care of and that he ought to get himself up and out the door.

Charlie confronts his greed very slowly. We have had many conversations about what his net worth means to him, and even more what he hopes it means to others, most especially his mother. We understand the "freedom" it gives him. We have explored how his mother was insatiable in her financial desires, how she was always extremely critical and shaming of his father, and how Charlie was the chosen savior. It has been very difficult for Charlie to give up the illusion that his balance sheet can both protect him from self-hate and criticism and also entitles him to special care. In unconscious defense, Charlie hopes that merging with his net worth will protect him from feeling anxious. Of course, it doesn't and can't, so he keeps coming to therapy and, together, we face and slowly transform these very unacceptable aspects of himself.

I realize that I have written extensively about Klein's conceptualization of the negative emotions, so I must note that she was clear that through her depressive position, love and the capacity to love are also present from the first year of life. Over time, the baby realizes that the hated, envied one also is the needed, loved one and this realization leads to great guilt and the need to repair. When things go well, this cycle is repeated over and over, consolidating the self and other as whole and separate, good and bad. She was clear that love forms the core of the self (Klein & Riviere, 1964).

Projective identification

Projective identification is a spectacularly difficult concept for our rational, logical minds to encompass. It is an unconscious or phantasy process and is one way of looking at the complexity of intimate relationships, whether in the family or in psychotherapy.

Klein took Freud's concept of projection a step further. She theorized that the infant needs to get rid of the discomfort of bad feelings and, in his phantasy, he puts those feelings into another. The infant puts feelings into the (m)other so she can take care of both him and the feelings (Mitchell & Black, 1995). We need the concept of projective identification as long as our theory is

Projection

Freud outlined several ways the ego protects itself from emotional upset. Projection is among his original ideas. According to this idea, we each have beliefs, attributes, and attitudes that we do not consciously identify with but may see or "project" onto others. For example, I might believe you are contemptuous of me, and the reality is that I am unconsciously contemptuous of you. Projection is the source of the universal ability to create "others" who are not like me and therefore dangerous to me.

"one-person"—you live in your skin and mind and I live in my skin and mind, and our boundaries are pretty fixed. So, if the baby is upset—hungry, cold, frightened, or angry—the mother "finds herself" upset as well. In Kleinian theory, in one-person psychology, the baby has put the upset onto his mother in order to get her to do something and make his life better. The baby is communicating as best he can, through emotion and action, and the mother is receiving as best she can. It is an important form of primitive communication between two separate people. That is, it is communication through emotions and actions not words. Hopefully, the mother is not nearly as upset as her baby and can find ways to calm both of them.

In the therapeutic situation, a parallel process occurs. If a patient is distressed, that upset is communicated nonverbally, and the analyst experiences herself as changed by the interaction between them. In Klein's mind projective identification is a negative occurrence—it is primitive, maybe even a hostile act on the part of the patient towards the analyst. To my mind, this kind of emotional exchange happens between people all the time. As a therapist, I see it as my job to allow this process, like any unconscious process, to become more conscious and develop into a source of information and progress. In today's world it is referred to as an enactment and will be discussed in great detail in Chapter 7.

For example, as I am waiting for Suzi to come to the door, I feel centered and expectant. However, the moment she crosses my threshold, I become unaccountably anxious. What happened? In the one-person world of Melanie Klein, Suzi put her anxiety into me and I allowed it to enter my being. From a strictly Kleinian perspective, Suzi has unconsciously, aggressively attacked me and now I must deal with that nonverbal communication. Without an awareness of the process of projective identification, I might wonder what has happened inside of me to create this inner disturbance. Is my sudden change of inner state strictly mine, or did it come from her? My job is to be aware of my personal reactivity to what I have taken in. Then, I must digest it and find a way to talk about it with Suzi. Through this helpful concept, I can entertain the notion that Suzi is anxious and that I am the recipient of her mood. Suzi does not consciously mean to make me anxious. She may not even realize how anxious or distressed she is. Her distress is too much for her to bear and she needs to "share" it, give some away. She is communicating nonverbally what she cannot yet fully translate into words.

Today, we have come to understand that projective identification—a very real, observable experience—is not a matter of putting one set of feelings into another person. We now understand that this kind of exchange is an ongoing, human limbic and right-brain communication. We "read" each other all the time. We will find in the chapters to come that this process is continuous, pervasive, and protective. It is key to our ability to connect and be understood.

Klein made many contributions to analysis and therapy and offered alternative notions and perspectives to the classical Freudian theories. While Freud had hoped that his concept of ego could fully manage id impulses, Klein maintained that we stay always complex, multi-layered, and less linear. The Freudian model maintained that the amount of energy or libido is limited and fixed. Klein came to believe there was no conservation of energy: the principles of both love and aggression keep expanding. Crucially, she moved the possibility of help and healing back into the first year of life, with a focus on an infant's formative first relationship, the mother or another primary caregiver. For Freud, the key parent was the father, the target of Oedipal rivalry and the source of rules and, therefore, guilt. Klein's descriptions of positions pictured our psychic worlds as fluid throughout life. Under stress, we can all revert to our more primitive selves. Her focus on the more painful protective emotions of greed and envy invite us to address these in ourselves and in others. Finally, the concept of projective identification opened psychotherapy to becoming more transactional, less isolated, less contained, and theoretically objective. I feel tremendous gratitude to Klein for noticing and naming all these very difficult and complex aspects of being human, even as I disagree with her explanations for these aspects of our nature.

There are many important theoreticians that emerged from the Kleinian tradition. I will discuss the three very different men who have helped me the most clinically: Wilfred Bion from the British school, and Otto Kernberg and Thomas Ogden from the American school.

WILFRED BION

Wilfred Bion (1897–1979) had a difficult, even traumatic, life. Born in British colonial India, he was sent away to England for schooling at age eight, never to return. Then he went straight from prep school to military tank service in World War I, where his "soul died" (Bleandonu, 1994). From our vantage point of today, he clearly suffered from PTSD, possibly sensitizing him to the vicissitudes of dissociation and psychotic anxieties, topics he deeply understood. Post university he became a medical doctor, practicing as a psychiatrist. During World War II, he served as a doctor to traumatized soldiers. Tragically, his wife died during childbirth and he was left with a baby daughter to raise. It was not until World War II was over that he undertook a full training analysis with Klein, became a psychoanalyst, and also married for a second time.

Bion is fiendishly difficult to read and I am indebted to Grotstein's (2007) interpretations and explications. Bion wants to convey non-dual ideas in words, and words always create duality: this, not that. At the time he was practicing and writing, the Eastern concept of non-duality was not part of Western thinking. Today, there are many non-dual teachers all advocating that within "ultimate reality" we are "all one" and on other planes of being, the "I–other" is no more. Grotstein refers to Bion as a mystic, not in the religious sense, but in the sense of becoming at one with and directly knowing a higher order of life.

Bion enjoins us to not only deeply "know" our patients, but also to become one with the patient, tolerating all the uncertainty that comes from this stance. So, when Bion writes that psychoanalysis is about the transformation from O to K, he is pointing to the non-dual transformation of "absolute impersonal knowing" to the knowledge of personal reality. Hard to read and understand, harder still to embody. According to Grotstein, once the analytic community began to understand Bion's injunctions, training had to change. A theory of pathology and a technique of change was not enough. Rather, the analyst needs to be able to enter the state of being called "reverie" by Bion and patiently contain all that comes, tolerating anxiety and uncertainty and not-knowing. Again, in Grotstein's words, the analyst has to move beyond both the paranoid-schizoid and the depressive position to a transcendent position (Grotstein, 2007).

Bion's theory of thinking involved the need to change "beta elements" or psyche-soma experience into "alpha elements"—that is, the awareness and capacity to think thoughts. Bion did not suggest such elements literally exist; rather, he is giving language to complex and multi-layered processes generated by the human mind and emotions (Bleandonu, 1994). Bion maintained that this is how we learn to "think," by gathering tolerance to frustrations, learning to wait to have our needs met.

For decades, Bion stayed on the edges of psychoanalysis because of how abstract his concepts are. Yet, now, some of those same concepts are mainstream, specifically the container ↔ contained, and the ability to be in reverie. Bion (1962) proposed that the infant needs the presence of a mature mind in order to help him consolidate his reality from a continuous stream of beta elements or sensations. The mother "contains" and "digests" the swirl of affects in her baby, then gives them back to him in a "digested" or thinking form. In Kleinian thinking, this is an example of projective identification. The mother becomes the container of the baby's bits and pieces. Container ↔ contained are each part of the other. We need two words to talk about them, but the overall idea points to one lived experience.

Bion is describing what the mother does as she approaches her upset baby and says with a rhythmic, melodic voice, "There, there; everything is going to be all right," communicating to the babe that he is understood. Someone is with him and the "bad" that is happening can become "good." It is not the words but the melody that contains and digests his upsets. The song in his mother's voice lets him know things are OK; Bion defined this maternal reverie as the mother's capacity to make sense of what is going on inside the babe (Bleandonu, 1994). She has transformed beta elements into alpha elements in Bion language. One way I think about reverie is that it is an act of faith in unconscious process; mothers don't know explicitly how they will take care of each upset, but they trust that they can and will. Therapists never know what will unfold in each session but must trust that something will happen that will benefit the growth of the patient.

As the therapist, if I sit in reverie—containing my own anxieties and resisting the desire to make concrete, helpful suggestions—then I can give back a reflection, a contained or digested reworking of our shared anxiety. The other is not alone, and the phenomena of the moment can become manageable.

To be with Jess, I quiet myself, patiently watching and waiting for her words. Jess needs a lot of spacious time to find words that express her inner experiences. Her mother and her husband are very quick with words, throwing out ideas and questions at a pace that Jess experiences as an attack. Historically, her response has been to panic internally when around them, and then to either become withdrawn or rageful. She has lost track of her dreams and she struggles to connect with the positive in her life. Her husband is quick to point out all that is good in their lives. On an objective level, he is right. Yet, Jess is struggling with very personal losses around the hopes she has cherished for herself at this time of her life. Because all is good on the outside, Jess does not feel entitled to her inner feelings of disappointment and dismay. Because of this, she needs a lot of space and time to find the words to express what is troubling her. She feels shame at how "slow" she is at finding her words, so this shame is an additional barrier to expressing herself. We sit together and breathe together. I communicate to her that it is fine to wait for her words to emerge. Occasionally, I will ask a question based on what I see in her face, hoping to open the feelings just below the surface. Mostly, we sit in silence, comfortably waiting. I find Bion so helpful in sitting with Jess. He frames for me her inability to convert her inner experience into words, and, therefore, her need for space. Bion's reverie is the best way to be with Jess, to convey my faith in her and her way of being in the world.

The capacity to hold opposites as part of the creative tension of life fascinated Bion. According to him, we both desire knowledge and refuse to know it when knowledge of reality is too painful. Then we "break the link" and refuse to know. Like Klein, Bion felt that a part of each of us is psychotic—that is, non-rational and impulse- and affect-driven, no matter how healthy we become—and that we are always in a fluid state of development, able to regress as well as progress (Bion, 1959, 1990).

Importantly, Bion elaborated Klein's concept of projective identification, considering it to be a threefold event: a communication, a form of defense, and a form of containment (Mitchell & Black, 1995). In Bion's world, the analyst and the patient are fundamentally far more enmeshed than in the classical tradition. We might even write patient ↔ analyst. Projective identification is now more interpersonal, and the analyst is always resonating with and wanting to contain both the patient's anxieties and his own. The Freudian idea of scientific objective knowing is no longer possible.

When Suzi is very anxious and upset, she "communicates" nonverbally and I feel it with her. That is one part of the story. A second aspect of the event is that Suzi uses anxiety to defend against something that is hidden from her consciousness, a dark feeling that is even more difficult to bear. The two of

(continued)

(continued)

us will need time and focus in order to find out what else is going on at this deeper level. My hypothesis is that, underneath her anxiety, she feels terribly empty and lonely. From a third perspective, Suzi is doing her best to contain these utterly unbearable feelings by sharing her upset with me through her contagious anxiety.

Over time, Bion came to focus on the phenomenology of what happened between him and his patient moment by moment. His famous injunction to other analysts to start each session "without memory, desire, or understanding" is a very difficult injunction to follow (Mitchell & Black, 1995). It opens the analyst/therapist to the unknown of his own feeling life. For him, this was the best way to be truly present to each unfolding moment—to be immersed in the phenomenology between doctor and patient. Bion argued that emotional experience is the foundation for both mental development and the search for truth. He had faith that the spontaneous emotional truth of any moment would engender healing.

Paradoxically, Bion also wanted analysis to become more scientific, even mathematical, and made many attempts at creating formulas to describe what he was talking about, which are very difficult to follow. His language embraces such ideas as the "ineffable," or the "unknowable," or the "ultimate Truth." Exquisitely he spoke of needing to know Truth with our inability to find Truth. Late in life, he wrote that existence is not enough, for existence must also have aliveness. I take both of these ideas to be statements from his direct knowing of the non-dual world (Grotstein, 2007).

As I have already noted, in Bion's mature writings, the analyst and the patient are fundamentally intertwined—a very different stance from the original Freudian/Kleinian view of two very separate minds. Thus, I can write patient ↔ analyst, although Bion certainly did not. In Bion's imagination, his patient was not revealing his mental contents to a neutral analyst. Rather, the patient experienced the analyst as different at every meeting, almost a different analyst depending on the emotional connection and the patient's inner world. He would refer to the statement of Heraclitus that you can't step into the same river twice (Grotstein, 2007). For Bion, both analyst and patient live in a world of hope and dread, and each meeting is potentially an emotional thunderstorm. The analyst must resonate with and contain both the patient's anxiety and their own anxiety and knows they can be unbalanced and upset by the patient. According to Bion, all analysis is an interaction between two different personalities, both subject to pressures—inside and out—each with defenses and dependencies. These two people are continually responding to every moment in the situation. Each is a human being within the commitment to privilege the patient's inner life as the leading edge and guide of all conversations. Without naming it as such, Bion wrote as a two-person theorist from a non-dual, transcendent position.

OTTO KERNBERG

Otto Kernberg is the most prominent contemporary American psychiatrist in the Freudian/Kleinian lineage and he could not be more different from Bion both personally and theoretically. His mind is an organizing mind, and he has systematized and updated classical theory, integrating it with Kleinian object relations and adding an important developmental layer. Kernberg was born in Vienna between the two world wars and his assimilated Jewish family fled Nazi Germany in 1939 to settle in Chile. There, he became a psychiatrist, and emigrated with his wife, to the East Coast of the US in 1959. He has contributed most profoundly to our understanding of borderline and narcissistic personality difficulties by considering both ego psychology and Kleinian object relations.

Kernberg's writings are rich and abstract. I am very indebted to both Mitchell and Black (1995) and J. Klein (1987) for their insights, summaries, and clarifications. In Kernberg's developmental model, there are three levels of pathology (Mitchell & Black, 1995). The first level contains psychotics, who have failed to establish the first developmental task of "me–not me." A psychotic does not know where any given thought originates: from inside, from the other person in the room, from the coffee pot? This level of development requires both medication and a safe environment in order to create any kind of life. At the second developmental level, the boundary of "me–not me" is clearer, but people at this stage cannot integrate hateful feelings and loving feelings for another person into a full, albeit ambivalent and complex human relationship. They are stuck at an infantile or split level of development—Klein's paranoid-schizoid position. They are often desperate for relationship, yet those relationships are full of pain and drama. They struggle to stay connected but explode regularly into anger, often violently turning away and leaving the relationship, seemingly forgetting the good when they connect with the bad. These are the "borderline and narcissistic" personalities, notoriously difficult to help and heal. At Kernberg's third level, neurotics have the classical Oedipal issues described by Freud, including an inability to deal with their intrapsychic conflicts. Nevertheless, they have self–object boundaries with good integration of positive and negative feelings. They are clearer that they can choose to fight or walk away and still stay connected.

Like Klein, Kernberg sees good and bad feelings as the fundamentals of vitality (Klein, J., 1987), creating a sense of self over time. In contrast to Freud, these discrete good and bad feelings are primary and formative; only later they become consolidated and eventually are experienced as drives. Subjectively registered good feelings and satisfying interactions become a pleasure-seeking drive. Subjectively registered bad feelings with unsatisfying interactions consolidate into an aggressive drive. These aggressive impulses are especially dangerous because they can be directed at others who also are loved.

By integrating Kleinian object-relations theories and ego psychology, Kernberg's developmental model begins earlier in life than the Freudian drive model. For him, the centerpiece of personality is the individual's developmental level of internal object relations, whether it be at a psychotic level, a borderline-narcissistic level, or a neurotic level (Mitchell & Black, 1995).

Love

Kernberg has a lot to say about sexuality and love connections. According to Kernberg, sexuality, the Freudian pleasure principle or libido, is not a direct cause of psychopathology. Rather the Kleinian earlier structures of self–object relationships create the meanings and enactments encoded within sexuality and these same object relations are the source of the difficulties. He further delineated sexuality and love within his framework of three levels (Mitchell & Black, 1995). At the most disturbed or psychotic level, relationships do not occur on a continuum, involving privacy and intimacy; either there is no relationship whatsoever or there is total merger. At the middle level of integration, the personality disorders that he is most interested in, sexual desire cannot be melded with intimacy and tenderness. Individuals operating at this level keep sexuality and intimacy split into separate categories. Moreover, passion might be infused with aspects of "not-me" for example, violence or disgust. At the neurotic level, both self and other are whole, and the difficulties arise over unconscious and misunderstood impulses rather than a complete splitting process as in his middle, or borderline-narcissistic, category. For him, these neurotic issues are still best understood in the classical drive tradition.

Treatment

For Kernberg (1975; 1984), the most fundamental problem at the middle level of development is innate and disavowed destructive aggression. Like Klein, he believes that narcissistic and borderline issues have a significant constitutional base, and that people with these issues have to construct defenses to protect themselves from becoming aware of their own capacity to hate both others and themselves. He outlines three levels of narcissism: normal adult, normal child, and pathological (Kernberg, 1975). Using his theoretical position of constitutional innate aggression, he integrates the Kleinian focus on the primitive destructive emotions and defenses, such as envy and greed, within this middle level of development, the narcissistic and borderline states of being.

He calls his method of therapy transference-focused psychotherapy and offers very specific insights into both the borderline and narcissist dilemmas. He notes that the borderlines typically use a great deal of splitting and idealization to keep their internal coherence while the more narcissistically inclined individuals idealize themselves and devalue others. As with Freudian and Kleinian analysis, his work is based on meeting several times a week working with the transference. His interpretations confront the defenses that borderline and pathologically narcissistic people employ in order to hold contradictory internal representations of themselves and their significant others. They are unable to employ the humanizing modulation of love and empathy to keep good connections. As these splits emerge in the transference, they are consistently confronted and interpreted by a very involved analyst, allowing integration to happen. Where the treatment differs from the traditional analytic frame is that there is a specific contract that holds both patient and clinician responsible to participate in specific ways, particularly around self-harm and other treatment-destroying tendencies of this middle group (Kernberg, 1984; 2015).

While Kernberg's is strictly a one-person model, he acknowledges that working with this middle group of individuals will often elicit strong reactions in the analyst, threatening his neutral stance (1975). However, he advocates using these reactions only and specifically as information about the patient, noting that chaotic and intense countertransference feelings imply more regression in the patient. It is critical that the analyst allow this process in order to stay in touch with the patient and at the same time not lose his own ego functioning both internally and if necessary use the external boundaries which are set by the process (capacity to hospitalize, groups, etc.).

Kernberg (2015) is keenly aware that in today's world of evidence-based treatments, psychoanalysis has not done enough research to further psychoanalysis as both a science and as a profession. He, himself, is doing research and imploring other psychoanalytic groups to do the same. His transference-based model for severe pathologies is now labeled evidence-based in an effort to prove it as effective, if not more so, as the cognitive behavioral methods which also claim that status.

> *Remember Mary, who has an autistic child and struggles with Kleinian envy? I often think of Kernberg when I sit with her. His focus on negative emotions and on the transference is exactly where our work unfolds. Her early history of emotional and physical abuse at the hands of her mother left Mary full of self-hate in spite of her professional accomplishments. Dealing with the envy, rage, and hate around her autistic son has re-awakened all of her early traumatic terror and rage. Mary finds it hard to believe that these violent feelings and impulses are normal for a terrified child, and that they need to be accepted before they can "grow up," evolve, and become a part of her. Although Mary cannot yet integrate her destructive aggression, she is deeply ashamed of it, acknowledging that she has "destroyed" her social relationships over the last few years. Mary is waiting for me to "get rid" of her, even though her concrete, personal experience of me is that I do not hate her in spite of all the horrible things she thinks and a few that she has done. Meanwhile, we continue to sort out the triggers that bring her destructive envy to the surface. Even though we have a long way to go, she reports less shame and social anxiety, and frankly marvels at my not "hating her as she deserves."*

THOMAS OGDEN

The other contemporary American who was strongly influenced by Klein is psychiatrist, essayist, and novelist Thomas Ogden. Based on the West Coast, Ogden (1986) wrote initially about Klein, Bion, and Winnicott and their impact on theory and practice of analysis helpfully enlarging and deepening our understanding of Klein's two positions and Winnicott's acceptance of paradox as part of the human condition.

Ogden (1989) then extended Klein's two positions—the paranoid-schizoid and the depressive—even further back in time to include what he named the autistic-contiguous mode of experiencing. This mode of being is totally sensory and in no way interpersonal. It involves bodily sensations as they interact with the world of both things and people. Like Klein, Ogden proposes that all three positions are modes of experiencing, each always available throughout life. We humans move among them depending both on the context and on internally generated feelings. Klein maintained that we are always in flux, our minds and states of being never fixed. Ogden further elucidated how each of these ways of being has its unique way of managing anxiety and different ways of relating to self and others. While sitting with his patients, he attunes to all three modes within the patient and himself. This fluidity is ongoing and never-ending.

Ogden's autistic-contiguous mode is a sensory, pre-symbolic way of generating experience, the foundation of the initial sense of inner place and self-experience. Sensory data creates a boundary at the surface of the skin, the rudimentary sense of "me–not me." It is through the skin that the baby experiences being held and nursed. Freud was very clear that the first ego is a body-ego. Ogden (1989) elucidates a much more refined picture of how that earliest sense of self develops in the rhythm of connection between mother and baby.

"Jack" frequently experiences himself as falling apart. When in this disorganized state, he talks in incomplete sentences, moving quickly between intense shame and incandescent rage. Bion helps me sense how Jack experiences himself in "bits and pieces," needing an outside container to hold, digest, and return something to him that he can use—my words, my care, our connections. Jack falls into a world of "beta elements," intense psyche-soma distress, and only through our being together can he find a calm place where he can both absorb his emotions and decide what to best do in his difficult life situation.

But it is Ogden's autistic-contiguous mode that is most useful in helping me to create the necessary container for Jack's feelings. When Jack experiences himself as falling apart, as being overwhelmed by too many feelings, I first direct Jack to his body as the sensory container of those feelings. Focusing on his body and his breathing, we enter Ogden's autistic-contiguous mode of experience, and access the ability to slow down the sensory stream and focus on a single sensation at a time. When we do this, Jack often spontaneously asks to lie on the carpet, needing to relax and be in contact with his whole body. With the help of Ogden's theory, I seek to move Jack from the paranoid-schizoid mode where everything is in bits and pieces—feelings and facts and self and other—to the container created by the concrete sensations of his body. This is the essence of Ogden's sensual autistic-contiguous mode. When we focus on his body and breath, Jack typically becomes aware of his chest region, his racing heart, and a sense of terror. By being together in this terrible bodily state, he has discovered how to slow down his breath and eventually calm himself. As he does this, Jack uncovers a paradox: For him, terror is always available, and, at this very moment, there is nothing to be frightened of. With this realization, we have a new possibility. We can move from Ogden's autistic-contiguous mode based on the sensations of the body to Klein's depressive mode, where there is a containing self that is capable of observing and thinking.

Ogden (2005) strongly emphasizes the patient's need to be known by the analyst and by himself and the analyst's need to know the patient. Ogden acknowledges true intersubjective knowing is complex, multi-layered, and very difficult. For me, he wants to live in the transitional space—for him, the dream space—of Bion's injunction that each meeting be fresh and new and at the same time learn about this patient and what this patient needs. Each dyad is unique, and each day is new. For him the analytic project has become that of increasing the patient's capacity to be alive, to tolerate the flow of human experience.

For me, Bion, Kernberg, and Ogden are part of Klein's lineage, all acknowledging her profound influence on both their thinking and practice. At the same time, each became quite different both from another and from Klein herself. Bion's increasingly interpretive and phenomenological approach focused on what he referred to as the thunderstorm that always occurs when two people interact. It seems to me he became less concerned with healing and more interested in noticing and living in the layers of complexity revealed within the examined life (Bleandonu, 1994).

Kernberg is closer to Klein with his more confrontational, one-person psychology intent on healing pathological developmental delays. Additionally, Kernberg is keenly aware that if psychoanalysis is to survive it must evolve and respond to the new information from brain science. Ogden, like Bion (whom he admires greatly), writes extensively about the interaction between analyst and patient and the uniqueness of each pair (Ogden, 1997). Both Bion and Ogden theorize within the framework of a two-person psychology, in which each pole of the dyad influences the other in continual exchange.

Kleinian theory and tradition moved our understanding of the human mind into deeper and more mysterious territory than the conflict and drive model of Freud. Both the Kleinians and other members of the British object-relations school used direct observation of infants and children to deduce the poignant truth, that for the tiny infant, an unmet need is a matter of life and death. Through experience and imagination, they further concluded that primitive rage and psychotic anxiety in certain adults can feel exactly the same—a matter of life and death. Thanks to modern neuroscience, we have a fuller understanding that in the first year of life the brain is unfinished, lending some objective weight to their subjective intuitions.

For Klein and Kernberg, these issues reside entirely within the patient. Like Freud, theirs is a clear one-person psychology. Bion and Ogden lean in the direction of a two-person psychology. They hold that each analysis is a unique, co-created relationship with the analyst holding a special responsibility to find the language and a way of being that will create ever-greater containers to heal the wounds of the past (Ogden, 1997).

Key concepts Chapter 3

Autistic-contiguous mode – Ogden's contribution to the Kleinian positions; refers to a sensory, bodily mode of being that underlies her two modes of experiencing

Bion's theory of thinking – the babe's beta elements, our earliest way of thinking is gradually transformed into alpha elements through interaction with another, more mature mind. Never considered "real," rather a way of thinking about thinking.

Contained – Bion's metaphor alluding to the baby's emotional/physiological needs in which beta upsets are transformed into alpha states

Container – Bion's metaphor for the mother's ability to manage her baby's upsets

Greed – wanting more than the other can give; one of Klein's core qualities of the newborn

Kleinian positions – idea that from the very beginning the babe can both "split" the world into good and bad and integrate the world into a more whole sense of you and me within the container of the mother

Manic defense – developed capacity to override painful feelings through action, discussed in great detail by both Klein and Winnicott

Neurotic level – a developmental achievement post-psychotic level wherein anxiety is managed through various defenses

Object – refers to the people who care for the baby allowing him to incorporate them or parts of them into his sense of self

One-person psychology – stance that each of us in maturity is solid and separate within our skin; in contrast to two-person psychology which suggests that we are all affecting each other all the time

Phantasy – Kleinian understanding of how the built-in drives of the babe are elaborated through unconscious experience early in life

Pre-Oedipal issues – all the archaic aspects of human life first outlined by the object-relations theorists where everything exists in an either/or state of being

Projective identification – first understanding of primitive bodily communication; how feelings from one person get into another before language

Psychotic level – a universal aspect of the human mind that exists before rational thought and the ability to manage emotional distress

Reverie – refers to first the mother's and then the therapist's ability to understand what is going on inside the other through using his own inner life

Split world – at the beginning the babe does not live in linear time, so each experience is discrete, creating a "good mother who takes care of me" paired with a "wonderful me" and a "bad mother who does not" paired with a "frustrated me"

References

Bion, W.R. (1959) Attacks on linking. In Spillius, E.B. (ed.) (1988) *Melanie Klein Today*. London: Routledge.
Bion, W.R, (1962) *Leaning from Experience*. New York: Basic Books.
Bion, W.R, (1990) *A Memoir of the Future*. London: Karnac.
Bleandonu, G. (1994) *Wilfred Bion: His Life and Works 1897–1979*. London: Free Association Books.
Brenner, C. (1955, 1974). *An Elementary Textbook of Psychoanalysis*. Garden City, NY: Anchor Press/ Doubleday.
Grosskurth, P. (1986) *Melanie Klein: Her World and Her Work*. New York: Knopf.
Grotstein, J.S. (2007) *A Beam of Intense Darkness: Wilfred Bion's Legacy to Psychoanalysis*. London: Karnac.
Kernberg, O. (1975) *Borderline Conditions and Pathological Narcissism*. New York: Jason Aronson.
Kernberg, O. (1984) *Severe Personality Disorders*. New Haven: Yale University Press.
Kernberg, O. (2015) Resistances and progress in developing a research framework in psychoanalytic institutes. *Psychoanalytic Inquiry*, 35: 98–114.
Klein, J. (1987) *Our Need for Others and Its Roots in Infancy*. London: Routledge.
Klein, M. (1957) *Envy and Gratitude*. London: Tavistock.
Klein, M. & Riviere, J. (1964) *Love, Hate and Reparation*. New York: Norton.
Mitchell, S. & Black, M. (1995) *Freud and Beyond*. New York: Basic Books.
Ogden, T. (1986) *The Matrix of the Mind*. Northvale, NJ: Jason Aronson.
Ogden, T. (1989) *The Primitive Edge of Experience*. Northvale, NJ: Jason Aronson.
Ogden, T. (1997) *Reverie and Interpretation: Seeing Something Human*. Northvale, NJ: Jason Aronson.
Ogden, T. (2005) *This Art of Psychoanalysis*. New York: Routledge.
Segal, H. (1979) *Melanie Klein*. New York: Viking.
Siegel, D.J. (2007) *The Mindful Brain*. New York: Norton.

4

ANNA FREUD

We have strengths as well as conflicts

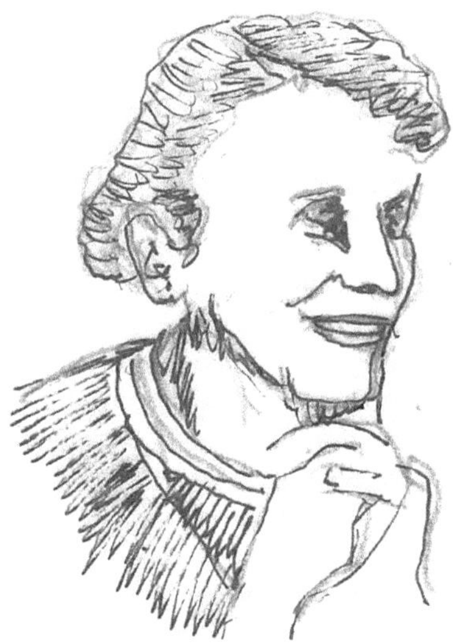

Anna Freud

Anna (1895–1982) was Freud's youngest child, and in later life she was emotionally and professionally closest to him. After being trained as a teacher, she decided to become an analyst, and, as was acceptable at the time, she underwent analysis with her father. Our thinking has evolved today; that would neither be acceptable nor viable. But it is helpful to remember that, in her time, the analyst was imagined as having a totally neutral, separate, and objective mind that could almost mechanically reflect back what was heard. Furthermore, as explained in previous chapters, the process of becoming an analyst consisted of being in analysis and then presenting a paper to the local psychoanalytic society. It wasn't until years later that organized institutes offering courses of study on analysis came along. Anna presented her first paper, which centered on beating fantasies and masturbation, to the Vienna Psychoanalytic Society in 1922. Of course, these are very "id" subjects, and presenting on such controversial topics was very courageous on her part (Young-Bruehl, 1988).

As noted previously, Freud had added the concept of an ego as a mediator between the id forces and the outer world. This was another step toward creating his tripartite model of id, ego, and superego. His original theory proposed that the id could not and did not learn. Therefore, the proposal of the ego suggested that, from the beginning, there was the potential of an inborn structure capable of learning and adapting. Freud's original id psychology (elaborated by Klein and her followers) was about taming raw sex and aggression. By 1936, Anna Freud was privileging the ego, celebrating and elaborating its capacity to both create and manage the id through inner mental structures called defenses. Ego psychology focuses on our capacity to learn, to adapt, and to create our individual sense of self, all the while acknowledging that the energy that fuels this project is the selfsame driving libido of the id. The ego psychologists find the mind to be inherently more stable, structured, and stratified than the terrified, always potentially chaotic landscape of the Kleinian positions. In the US, it is fair to say that traditional psychoanalysis belongs more to this lineage.

Anna published *The Ego and the Mechanisms of Defense* in 1936 in German. By focusing on the ego and its development, Anna elaborated our understanding of human character. She came to realize that, in the effort to make the unconscious conscious, the analyst was not only engaging with the intransigence of the presenting symptoms, but also the resistance of ego itself to reflection and awareness. The treatment developed by Anna became character analysis, with the goal of understanding the dynamic created in the crucible of the drives meeting the ego and the superego. She discovered that, paradoxically, the ego both wants to be free of suffering and also is dedicated to the protection of that same sense of self from unacceptable or unbearable insights. These two desires for freedom and safety are a constant balancing act, and defense mechanisms are created to maintain a manageable sense of identity. She catalogued the defense mechanisms we are all familiar with: projection, regression, sublimation, reaction formation, undoing, reversal, introjection, identification, and turning against the self. In her encounter with the ego defenses, Anna realized that, to free associate—the basic dictum of her father's form of therapy—was in reality very difficult. So, she framed it as a goal and achievement rather than expecting it as a straightforward capacity (Freud, A., 1936; 1966; 1935; 1960).

Anna was very much her father's daughter and it is perhaps too easy to say that she spent her life in his shadow, working constantly, wanting his approval, wanting to make meaningful contributions to psychoanalysis and wanting to have her own life, and be her own person. Like him, she constantly self-analyzed herself and used her dreams to guide her theories, not presenting them as hers, but rather as representations of the subject at hand. She analyzed the children of her friends, basing her theories on those limited experiences. In letters she acknowledged that she wished to have more from those children, especially the children of her close companion Dorothy Burlingham (Young-Bruehl, 1988). Clearly, she had a lot of conflicts and ambivalences to manage. She always acknowledged her father's sexual and aggressive urges as inherent in any child but contended that children were much more than just those urges. They needed creative and imaginative care to develop fully, to not be overly constrained by undue fear of authority, nor raised in a limitless atmosphere. She also engaged in proper research on a larger scale, using her various nurseries to present important findings on children and their developmental needs to the wider world (Solnit, 1986).

Anna's interest was always in children, first in Vienna and then in London. However, she was far less absorbed in the Kleinian world of the tiny baby with all its extreme vicissitudes and stark contrasts of life and death and the "good" and the "bad." Anna focused first on her father's Oedipal period and then on the later years of childhood, referred to as the post-Oedipal or latency period and adolescence. During this time, the child is concerned with gathering a self through learning about, mastering, and participating in the outer world. She wanted to understand normal, practical, everyday development and education and help both parents and educators raise emotionally healthy children (Freud, A., 1966). She focused on research, particularly with children deprived either by the turmoil of World War II or due to unfortunate or disrupted family circumstances (Freud, A. & Burlingham, 1943, 2015).

During the war, along with her partner Dorothy Burlingham, Anna founded first the Hampstead War Nurseries and, later, the Hampstead Clinic. These were lifelong projects that were dedicated to helping families and children, including disabled children, and training analysts to work with children. Many seminal publications came from their research, including some of the first on working with deprived, disabled, and blind children in an empathic and compassionate way. I find it sad that Anna referred to her love of research and writing as her penis-child, totally typical of the language of the time, but sad nevertheless (Young-Bruehl, 1988).

As part of her war nursery effort, over 1,000 children were brought from Europe and eventually placed and adopted in England and the US. I want to mention one special group of children that came to her attention and under the care of her organization. They were a group of six orphaned babies who had been attended to for three years by many caretakers in the concentration camp Theresienstadt. They arrived in London as a group and were found to be a very aggressive little gang, caring deeply for each other and only for each other. Their need to stay together was immediately recognized and they were given a home of their own in the north of England, along with consistent, well-trained caretakers. They were found to be remarkably healthy, confounding all the theories about needing a consistent, caring adult "other." They had formed a sibling group without the benefit of parents and seemingly without sibling competitions for that love. When writing about them, Anna noted that they were autoerotic, aggressive, restless, and difficult but were not in any way deficient, delinquent, or psychotic. By loving each other, they had mastered survival in a very unique way. Once given a consistent substitute mothering, they settled down, learned English, and their social and intellectual development continued. Truly an amazing story!

This little gang confirmed Anna's optimistic thesis that when given the opportunity to create good object relationships the aggressive drive could be appropriately fused with the libidinal drive—her father's language for sure (Young-Bruehl, 1988). This fueled her enthusiasm for the various nurseries she had established, which focused on the ego strengths of children and the research she was able to conduct in those settings.

Let's look at both Jess and Suzi through the lens of ego psychology and explore how differently they use ego defenses to help them through their struggles and conflicts. Jess' presenting symptom was depression "for no good reason." She knows that she has a very good life, including a good husband and a good job— Freud's love and work—yet she does not feel good or excited about her life. In her world, Jess is very high functioning, only at home does she regress and wish her mother and her husband would do something to make her feel better. She projects that they have the "power" to make a difference. In my office, Jess allows her anxieties about her slowness of speech to emerge. She reveals that her mother and her husband "speak very fast, and they know they are right." Furthermore, Jess also believes they are "right." There is nothing to be sad about, to wish were different. Jess abdicates her feelings and needs; she "turns against herself." When we sit together, she is free to take her time, to find her words and feelings, and honor herself in that way. Abdication protects her from conflict with the others, whom she deeply loves. However, she chronically feels "less than." Her defenses are not working for her and, at the same time, are very difficult to let go of and disturb the peace of the current system.

When I first met Suzi, I thought she had more robust ego defenses than Jess. Suzi felt alive, healthily entitled to speak her mind, and surer of herself. Like Jess, Suzi is very high functioning at work. However, when things go wrong, she will both deny and undo—often pretending that the outcome was what she intended when it clearly was not. It has taken many conversations to slow Suzi down, allowing her to find her feelings—of sadness, of regret, even occasionally of despair. Now, within our safe context, we can both acknowledge that her strengths, while real and helpful, cover some emptiness and loneliness.

Unlike Klein, Anna Freud maintained that when working with children, the child does not fall immediately into a transference relationship mimicking the child's relationship to his parents. She notes that the child still has his parents and now has someone new to relate to. So, for her, the relationship operates on both levels (Young-Bruehl, 1988). Anna had faith in the higher-functioning aspects of her patients, trusting that a relationship could be forged in the best interest of that part of the self.

Her research in post-war London illuminated childhood development from dependency to emotional self-reliance, bringing to the foreground the child's rapid mastery of skills, creative resolutions of conflicts, and the development of interests that further self-esteem (Freud, A., 1966). In contrast to Klein's terrified and desperate infant, Anna's theoretical baby is a robust, alive, learning creature, full of enthusiasm and possibility. Her developmental theory combined her father's drive theory with an emphasis on the importance of parents in creating the child's inner world, its object relations.

She wrote prolifically: research articles, clinical articles and letters to the entire analytic community on both continents. She enriched both psychoanalysis and early childhood education by deeply studying normal development. Her developmental theory was less stage-based and more continuous with the ongoing possibility of both forward and backward movement. She was very clear that the biological givens and the environment were in continuous interaction and both had to be considered. She was much more optimistic about resilience than either her father or Klein.

I need to mention one other important writing, "About losing and being lost," as mourning is such an important process in life. Here, she reflects on her own mourning processes in a profound and authentic way, differing somewhat from her father's understanding of the process already mentioned. In his writing, mourning can be complete. We can move on. Anna has a different experience, one certainly closer to my own. She acknowledges the human need to both stay loyal to the dead and create ties with the living. How to grieve and how to move on are critical human dilemmas, never solved and never settled, always visited and re-visited (Freud, A., 1967).

Anna Freud traveled to the US many times and was consistently well received there. She eventually became a foundational figure for American psychoanalysis and psychotherapy, making her emphasis on the capabilities of the ego the main thrust of that tradition.

HEINZ HARTMANN

Anna Freud had a number of important colleagues, who have become key thinkers in expanding our understanding of human nature and how to help people who are suffering. Heinz Hartmann (1894–1970) is considered by many to be the founder of ego psychology, as Anna is often considered too embedded in her father's thinking on the centrality of conflict. He was analyzed by Freud himself, but then had to escape Europe, emigrating to New York City in 1941. In 1937, he had written his foundational paper on the ego in German, envisioning a baby full of positive potentials ready to bloom in the right environment. Hartmann was deeply interested in the concept of mental health and continually focused on the adaptive, creative functions of the ego. He hypothesized the then radical idea that we each have within us a sphere that is without conflict. At the time, such a notion was utterly new to psychoanalysis (Mitchell & Black, 1995).

Like most analysts, Hartmann wanted to stay within the classical Freudian tradition and at the same time make his own contributions. In order to understand the importance of his particular contributions, let's briefly review Freud's original thinking. Maturity, or what Freud called "secondary process thinking," develops when the child is forced to resolve the conflict between his pleasure needs—"primary process thinking"—and reality. The child has to think and respond realistically to avoid the discomfort of mounting instinctual pressures. This model was the template for the classical technique: non-gratification and interpretive confrontations would reveal id pressures and, thereby, transform the id energy into reality functioning.

Hartmann moved the focus away from id drives to the idea that we each have the ego possibility of continually adapting, learning, and acquiring skills. Moreover, in addition to our id drives, we have innate ego roots, such as perception, thinking, language, and intentions. In his view, the baby is not just drifting along in a sea of either gratification or upset, but, rather, has all of these adaptive potentials built into his being. Hartmann's theoretical baby unfolds organically in a receptive environment. For him, the psychological is an extension of the biological, just as a mother must take biological care of a baby for that baby to develop psychologically. Of course, conflict is always a possibility, but Hartmann's focus became non-conflictual adaptive development. His model entails looking simultaneously at both the problem and the adaptations generated by the problem (Hartmann, 1964).

Freud had proposed sublimation as the source of energy for the higher cultural functions. For Freud, all of art and civilization is created by libido, the same id energy that is the source of sexual gratification. Hartmann viewed the process differently and proposed the term "neutralization," through which the ego strips the drives of their sexual and aggressive qualities (Mitchell & Black, 1995). Once again, the emphasis is on the power of the ego, its agency and capacity to manage the id.

Hartmann noted that adaptation develops not only in a linear fashion, but also via detours into unconscious fantasy, and he proclaimed this to be good and normal. We need the reality-based hopes and expectations of our parents as well as our own non-rational hopes and dreams. For him, all of this is part of love, part of being fully human. We are rooted in conflicts as well as aspirations (Hartmann, 1964). This represents a huge change from the Freudian/Kleinian tradition, where we are *only* conflict.

Strongly influenced by Anna's position on her father's work and the forced migration of Hartmann and others, for decades American psychoanalysis was more influenced by the ego tradition than the Kleininan tradition. Both classical Freudian conflicts and the tenets of ego psychology ground the American canon. Together they are optimistic and full of agency. They acknowledge our innate capacities to grow, create, adapt, problem solve, and find our personal way to connect with people and ideas, as well as art and literature. Interpretation and insight are thought to be curative. Ego psychology represents a stance taken by therapists, counselors, and educators that focuses on positive abilities as well as the drives or intense inner conflicts. If Freud and Klein represent the "push" of development, Anna Freud and the ego psychologists represent the "pull" of achievement.

I hold these principles in high regard as underlying truths, and they guide a lot of my work. However, I still need Klein's help to transform Mary's envy, Charlie's greed, and Jack's falling apart. I better understand these issues through Klein's notion of the positions that can shift a person's inner ground of being as radically as an earthquake and with similarly devastating effects. It would seem that some people have had their adaptive resources utterly trampled. They need much insight, safety, support, and guidance in order to risk taking a next step. Today we would call this developmental trauma, and I will discuss that in Chapter 7 especially the contemporary Bromberg.

Mary provides a good example of Hartmann's view of the clinical process. Mary struggles with the very Kleinian issue of envy. Remember, Mary has an autistic son who is very disabled, and she is embittered by those who have "normal" children. Mary feels overwhelmed by her envy and her angry expressions. She views herself as only bad, not worthy of friendships. However, as we unpack her week, we find numerous small gestures of kindness, usually phone calls or texts to people in her community who are suffering in some way. Mary can reach out to these people because they might be feeling worse than she feels. In these moments, she feels OK, not great, not loving, but OK. Together we can use those moments to anchor a sense of "okayness," seeking a balance between envy and okayness. Both exist in her. She can locate a felt sense of both in her body. Slowly, she has come to realize that envy is not her sole way of being, allowing her to aspire to create more moments of feeling OK.

RENÉ SPITZ

Like many others in this story, René Spitz (1887–1974) was born in Vienna, studied the work of Freud, moved first to France, and then, in 1939, emigrated to New York, intending to work with other researchers on the effects of childhood deprivation. He is another key figure in this shift in attention from the focus on the intrapsychic struggles of the baby to the interaction between the baby and environment.

Rather than theorizing from individual patients like most of his colleagues, in the 1940s, Spitz (1946a, 1946b) studied two groups of babies raised under difficult circumstances. One group had been raised in an orphanage, where the infants were kept in cribs and one nurse cared for seven children. The other group was raised in a prison nursery, where they were cared for both by their mothers and prison staff. When the babies were four months old, there was little discernible difference between the two groups. However, by age one, the differences were striking: The children in the orphanage failed to develop both intellectually and physically. They were less curious and playful and more subject to infections. By age two, only two of these orphaned children could walk and most could say only a few words. The children raised in the prison nursery showed development comparable to what was deemed "normal development" based on other studies.

With this study, Spitz confirmed what other researches also were indicating: Babies need extensive personal human care in order to develop. What made Spitz's study so very powerful was that, in 1952, he released a heartbreaking film showing the dramatically limited development of the children in the orphanage and other institutions, including hospitals. As a result, institutions around the world were forced to notice and begin to change policies regarding parental visits and contact. The harrowing images in the film had an impact far greater than the words alone could ever have. Today, we have some understanding of the right brain's power to create feelings and heart-to-heart connections through images not words. But for now, I want to flag the impact: to watch this film is to be horrified and convinced that something different has to be done.

Spitz, as a classically trained analyst, believed that the libido of the child was focused on pleasure (the id drive), but his research added the invaluable idea that along with the need for pleasure was the developing ego need to care and be cared for by a specific other (Mitchell & Black, 1995). Spitz believed that each child creates his own "libidinal object," reflecting a specific attachment to a specific other. He highlighted Hartmann's principles of ego adaptation and reciprocal influence. The infant is not only moving through the Freudian developmental stages of oral, anal, to phallic discharge but is, at the same time, creating internal structures through that specific relationship with a specific caregiver. Spitz maintained that every aspect of early psychic development is mediated through the maternal environment, and to be deprived of that specific care, therefore, is devastating (Spitz, 1965).

Two additional concepts generated by Spitz are very important to me. "Anaclitic depression" refers to the child's reaction of grief, anger, and finally apathy when deprived of a loved and loving one for three months or less. This partial deprivation can be recovered from, albeit very slowly (Spitz, 1946b). The second is "hospitalism," or failure to thrive (Spitz, 1946a). This refers to the total deprivation of the loved one for a longer period. In these cases, he writes that the consequences are irreparable in infants and extremely difficult to overcome in older babies. Well-being is compromised because the infant can no longer depend on or trust in the environment. This results in the so-called schizoid factors more fully discussed in Chapter 5.

Studies done and undone

It is true that by today's standards, Spitz's work would not stand up to the rigors of the scientific method. Thank goodness his basic ideas were totally vindicated by a subsequent World Health Organization publication meticulously compiled by Mary Ainsworth (1962).

Jack suffers from the lack of such a specific caring relationship. He was raised by a series of nannies. His parents were distant and sometimes scary. In the Ogden section, I described how, when Jack "falls apart," he cries and shakes and sometimes can't get out of bed. At such moments, any organized sense of a self with agency and ongoingness is totally lost. Jack's history is not equivalent to the babies documented by Spitz; nevertheless, his very complex nature, composed of sparkling creativity undermined by intense terror, exhibits what happens to a human baby when he is deprived a specific caregiver, creating a specific relationship that can be internalized.

MARGARET MAHLER

While Spitz was writing and carrying on his important research, another figure arrived in New York after fleeing the war in Europe. Hungarian-born Margaret Mahler (1897–1985) had trained as a physician in Germany before becoming an analyst in Vienna. In 1938, she emigrated to New York, where she created a training/teaching institute as well as a private practice in both New York and Philadelphia (Smith, 1986). During this time, she, along with colleagues Fred Pine and Anni Bergman, conducted many studies of children, observing what happened between them and their mothers, and developed what became known as the separation-individuation theory of childhood development (Mahler et al., 1975). She documented her careful observations and interpreted what she saw through the one-person lens of analytic theory. Her language is focused on the intrapsychic not the interpersonal. Her empirically based observations of normal children within normal families is among the first truly scientific studies of its kind and a very different process from reconstructing history through the dreams and free associations of an adult patient.

Separation-individuation theory

In Mahler's model, development takes place in phases and over time. In the first iteration of her theory, the first few weeks of life are referred to as the "normal autistic phase," a nod to Freud's earliest, most primitive sense of oceanic oneness, during which the baby is rather detached and disconnected from the outer world and spends most of its time sleeping. Based on further research, she abandoned this phase in later papers. However, it has a place in developmental thinking because it is used in the first editions of her seminal book, *The Psychological Birth of the Human Infant*, required reading for students of both psychoanalysis and childhood development (Mahler et al., 1975).

Mahler's second phase is called the "normal symbiotic phase." During this stage, the child experiences herself as part of the mother. Child-and-mother are a special unit separate from the rest of the world, in a kind of paradise of union.

The individuation process

The individuation process is a phrase used in various ways in many traditions. A central feature for all is the idea that each individual must find his own distinct, separate, and unique identity, while at the same time remain connected to family and culture. This is the process that Abraham Maslow called self-actualization, a central tenet of humanistic psychology. Self-actualization refers to the process of becoming as fully whole and true to oneself as possible (Maslow, 1968).

At five to six months of age, the child begins to find or create his own individuality. This begins the "separation-individuation phase" composed of many phases or steps. "Separation" refers to the gradual letting go of the felt experience of "mommy and I are one." On the other hand, "individuation" refers to the development of the baby's personal sense of self or ego or individuality through the development of thinking abilities, including self-reflection. Both are needed to create that part inside each of us that we think of as "me." Both these strands—separation and individuation—are critical in Mahler's understanding of child development. The earliest part of this phase, when the baby emerges from her shell and is increasingly alert to the world, she referred to as "hatching." This is followed by the onset of motor development and the intensely physical "practicing phase" of the separation-individuation process. The child first turns over, then crawls, and then walks and runs. With each new motor achievement, she increases the possible distance between herself and her mother, discovering a wider world to explore. Mahler observed that many children have an exuberant increase of excitement and mobility around their first birthday, a phenomenon she referred to as a "love affair with the world." For these months, their energy is seemingly unbounded, and they are surprisingly resilient to minor bumps and scrapes (Mahler et al., 1975; Kaplan, 1978).

Around the middle of the second year of life, the babe enters what Mahler and her co-authors call the "rapprochement phase," and harassed mothers refer to as the "terrible twos." The babe is no longer satisfied with being able to move around and manipulate the external environment. Now he turns his focus—with great intensity—on the caregiver, alternately wanting her close, or harshly pushing her away; sometimes wanting to share everything with her, sometimes ignoring her completely. Mahler's hypothesis is that, at this stage, the baby realizes that his physical mobility means he is psychically separate from his mother and therefore endangered—what is called abandonment or separation anxiety. Each mother–baby pair must come to its own solution regarding optimal distance and optimal togetherness. Each member of the pair will proffer their own needs and preferences to their joint solution; therefore, this is a very tender and formative period. It seems likely that many patterns of dependency and intimacy are rooted here, during the second and third years of life.

Mahler's separation-individuation model is important not just for students of child development and psychoanalysis, but also for therapists and healers of all kinds. There are many parallels between a child's behavior during rapprochement and that of an adult who is struggling with dependency and autonomy, or borderline and/or narcissistic issues within adult relationships. Having a developmental model in mind, therapists can be more helpful to such individuals. Regression to an earlier phase of development, specifically the rapprochement time, has been among the most favored understandings of borderline and narcissistic issues (Masterson, 1981). In working with these patients, Mahler's framework makes more sense to many therapists than the Kleinian idea of a paranoid-schizoid position. Both point to similar phenomena of non-rational, non-logical ways of being in the world.

If I look at envy-ridden Mary through Mahler's developmental model, I can see her as the deeply ambivalent rapprochement baby who has not developed a part of adult self to moderate and modulate her distress. Like the two-year-old, when Mary is angry and upset, she has no access to other ways of being. In a triggered moment, she loses self-awareness. Each of us can "fall" into these regressed states with sufficient provocation. We all can "lose ourselves" in anger, abandonment anxiety, fear, or other negative states. For Mary, this is a frequent event, happening in every social situation where children are mentioned.

Mary's mother was unreliable and verbally abusive. Her father was unavailable both emotionally and physically. It is easy for me to imagine that when little Mary needed help to manage her intense feelings as a toddler, no one was forthcoming. I imagine that she was consigned to the realm of the "bad," with no hope of building a more integrated state. In her current life, she has had to contend with a starkly difficult situation. Anyone with a disabled child needs help to find the resources to meet this situation—especially Mary, for whom the alternative is believing the old story told to her by her mother that she is worthless and does not deserve to have good things in her life. Her child has become the out-picturing of her unworthy self.

ERIK ERIKSON

My next important name in the ego psychology lineage is Erik Erikson (1902–1994), yet another person who considered himself a neo-Freudian while at the same time modifying Freudian theory virtually beyond recognition. Erikson was analyzed by Anna Freud. He trained to be a child analyst, and like so many others, had to leave Germany in 1933. However, his early years also were significantly different from all of the thinkers in this book. He was born out of wedlock and adopted by his stepfather. He never knew his biological father and, arguably as a result of this, he spent his twenties wandering around Europe, feeling displaced in any country and disconnected from any religion. In searching for his own identity, he named himself, Erik Son of Erik. Once he arrived in Boston, he became the first official child psychoanalyst in the US—a self-appointed position. Despite having limited formal education, Erikson taught at many top universities, contributing to anthropology, ego psychology, and longitudinal research on human development (Mitchell & Black, 1995).

Erikson is perhaps best known for his seminal publication *Eight Ages of Man*, which tracks human development from birth through old age (Erikson, 1950). In Erikson's view, each of the eight stages he enumerates has a developmental task leading to various potential outcomes, positive and negative. These stages are psychosocial, rather than entirely intrapsychic—a very non-Freudian position. Moreover, he believed we could get derailed anywhere along the trajectory of life. Early childhood might be good, but adolescence traumatic. For example, if we fail to connect with meaningful love and work in young adulthood, the rest of life can be compromised. Erikson maintained that each of us must hold and then integrate the opposing tensions encoded in each life-stage challenge. Only by integrating the polar opposites of each stage—an arduous task—will we create the most fulfilling outcome. Erikson coined the phrase "identity crisis" to describe the effort required to hold these tensions at each stage, and he believed that life is a series of such crises.

Here are Erikson's stages across the life cycle, including their best outcomes:

- basic trust vs. mistrust, first year of life: identity and realistic hope;
- autonomy vs. shame, early childhood: will and determination;
- purpose and initiative vs. guilt, pre-school years: sense of purpose;
- competence and industry vs. inferiority, elementary school years: competence;
- fidelity and identity vs. role confusion, adolescence: capacity for connection and self-reflection;
- intimacy vs. isolation, young adulthood: ability to form nurturing, committed relationships;
- generativity vs. stagnation, later adulthood: capacity to love and work;
- ego integrity vs. despair, age 65 on: wisdom not bitterness.

Erikson's last two stages of development are lifelong adult issues that every sentient being faces. All adults have experienced disappointments and regrets and how those are internalized and managed makes a huge difference to well-being and quality of life. Bitterness is always an option when we feel we have been treated unfairly and have not gotten what we wanted from life. To contain those negative, painful experiences and transform them into wisdom is a lifelong project.

Erikson changed the psychoanalytic vocabulary. For him, the notion of drives is de-emphasized, replaced by concepts such as identity, hope, purpose, and wisdom (Erikson, 1950, 1968). These are all existential themes that move the idea of what is a human being away from the strictly biological natural sciences into something broader and more metaphysical.

Working within this foundation, others have enriched our understanding that development continues throughout life, although early childhood development is still considered crucial and formative. For example, with my patient Mary, her struggle with envy is rooted in a childhood marred by a verbally abusive mother. Anyone would find caring for a disabled child difficult, but Mary's escalation of her situation into a hate-ridden ordeal, casting her out of all her social circles, indicates a terrible legacy from her past. Before Erikson, it was assumed that development was complete by puberty. Thereafter, it was thought that our inner world is set and only the intense work of psychoanalysis could change what was formed. Within this view, there was no natural ongoing development in adult humans. We could continue to learn new things, but we did not develop internally and organically. Today, we acknowledge the neuro-plasticity of the brain even into old age (Siegel, 2007). We always can grow and develop and many of us want to. The greater consciousness proposed and sought after by the great spiritual traditions depends on this ever-spiraling possibility.

Finally, Erikson (1950, 1968) advocated a more complex, even benign approach to human aggression. To his mind, we need to understand that the original Freudian drive of aggressiveness is used first to fuel motility and then agency, the capacity to move and create on our own behalf. These forms of aggression are growth-enhancing, not destructive or hostile.

Erikson's work inspires me for it proclaims that personal development is always possible, there are unknown and important aspects of life to be uncovered, lived, and reflected upon throughout life. For Erikson, it is never too late to become more curious about oneself, life, and others. Change is always possible (Erikson, 1950, 1968).

I find it valuable to have a developmental model across the life span when working with anyone who is engaged with or questioning life's meaning. When the marriage is successful, when the kids are launched, when there is enough job security or money in the bank, what is there left to do? How can I "be" in the second half of life in a fulfilling way? Erikson's concept of generativity is a spectacularly helpful guiding principle. Many people enter therapy with some form of "mid-life depression." Understanding that there is a "pull" to become more, not just the "push" of earlier pathology sets a fresh and life-enhancing tone, allowing each of us to discover our personal ways of giving, participating, and interacting with the wider world.

Although there are other important names in the lineage of the ego psychoanalysts, those offered here represent the important developments in England and the US during and after World War II. It might appear from these brief synopses of their lives and work that they were unaware of each other. Of course, this is not true. The world of psychoanalysis has always been small, and in the 1940s, 1950s, and 1960s, everyone knew everyone else, at least in a peripheral way. All were influencing each other and talking to each other through papers and conferences. This will become clearly apparent when considering Winnicott and the middle or independent school.

During this time, using the transference to uncover the unconscious and understanding the resistances was still the centerpiece of analysis (Greenson, 1967). The patient tries to get gratification from the analyst and the analyst interprets those archaic desires. For the ego psychologists, transference is augmented by the working alliance between analysts and patient. Whatever unconscious repetition is being enacted was understood as the arena where we each continue to attempt to build normal psychic structures. From this perspective, transference is no longer only a problem to be solved. It is a universal phenomenon to be understood, to be deeply and respectfully curious about. The analyst is trying to understand which aspects of psychic structure have been compromised through a verbal exchange and then seeks to discover which can be repaired. The experience between analyst and patient is an opportunity to understand both the nature of the patient's disruptions and his efforts to compensate for those disruptions and failures. Within this context, the patient can then use the analysis to rework and repair these missing places and indirectly fulfill unmet needs (Mitchell & Black, 1995).

Freud's metaphors were of excavating and war. The classical analyst must dig underneath the presented narrative to find the deeper truth. The ego psychologists added the phrase working alliance within a metaphoric partnership (Greenson, 1967). They believed that the very fabric of psychic structure was first consolidated within a human partnership. Therefore, each of us always needs a continuous, subtle, empathic tie to another in order to modify that old tie. Growth happens as we modify that old arrangement, allowing a fuller or at least less constricted life. Nevertheless, all of the ego psychologists considered themselves to be within the Freudian lineage. This is still the world of one-person psychology, where there is an authority that knows and stays "neutral" within that subtle tie and a patient who is the sole source of all problematic issues.

When I wrote of Bion and Ogden, I spoke of Jess as a case of silently sitting and patiently waiting to see what would emerge. The ego psychology tradition, with its emphasis on resilience despite obstacles and its faith in continuous development, also is a good frame for Jess. She needs a lot of space and a lot of time, but it is clear that she has everything she needs to create her next steps from within herself. She proffers her own unique ideas about how to proceed, when to confront her husband, and how to talk to her mother. She can access pleasure in spite of some physical limitations and losses. Jess can think about herself and use her imagination to visualize her future. In the Erikson model, she is becoming generative, rather than stagnating as she discovers new options in spite of real limitations.

Key concepts Chapter 4

Abandonment or separation anxiety – the intense panic experienced when separated from the mother for too long; now considered the source of much psychological suffering in adults

Anaclitic depression – the normal emotional response of grief and anger of a child who is separated from his caring others for three months or less

Generativity – Erikson's term for the best of adult development, the capacity to create, find meaning, and give back

Hospitalism – the apathy or failure to thrive a child falls into when separated for too long from those he needs and depends on

Individuation process – the normal growth pattern of decreasing dependence on the caring others as the excitement of exploration develops

Libidinal object – the good each baby both creates and discovers in his caring other

Mid-life depression – Erikson noted that many people suffered a loss of meaning and depressed affect when they had accomplished their material or conscious goals

Neutralization – Hartmann's concept that the ego could reduce the power of the id drives, rather than sublimate or re-direct that power as Freud proposed

Normal autistic phase – Mahler's first phase of development; later renamed as her research demonstrated that the neonate is always relational, never self-contained

Normal symbiotic phase – Mahler's term for the second stage of development during which the baby is believed to experience himself as often merged with the mother or caring other

Rapprochement phase – Mahler's term when the two-year-old discovers the conflict between his desire to be separate and his desire to be connected

Reciprocal mutual influence – Hartmann's idea that the baby and the mother are affecting each other and need each other; continually important to both self psychology and relational psychology

Separation-individuation phase – with mobility, the toddler begins to explore her world still needing the secure base of the mother

Separation-individuation theory – Mahler's developmental theory based on direct observations of mother–child pairs

Working alliance – the phrase the ego psychologists used to describe the relationship between analyst and patient

References

Ainsworth, M.D.S. (1962) The effects of maternal deprivation: A review of findings and controversy in the context of research strategy. In *Deprivation of Maternal Care: A Reassessment of Its Effects*. Public Health Papers No. 14. Geneva: World Health Organization.

Erikson, E. (1950) *Childhood and Society*. New York: Norton.

Erikson, E. (1968) *Identity: Youth and Crisis*. New York: Norton.

Freud, A. (1935, 1960) *Psychoanalysis for Teachers and Parents*. Boston: Beacon.
Freud, A. (1936, 1966) *The Ego and the Mechanisms of Defence*. London: Hogarth.
Freud, A. (1966) *Normality and Pathology in Childhood*. London: Hogarth
Freud, A. (1967). About losing and being lost. *Psychoanalytic Study of the Child*, 22 (1): 9–19.
Freud, A. & Burlingham, D. (1943, 2015) *War and Children*. Philadelphia: Great Library Collection. Originally published by the Foster Parents' Plan.
Greenson, R.R. (1967) *The Technique and Practice of Psychoanalysis*, vol. 1. New York: International Universities Press.
Hartmann, H. (1964) *Essays on Ego Psychology*. New York: International Universities Press.
Kaplan, L. (1978) *Oneness and Separateness: From Infant to Individual*. New York: Simon & Schuster.
Mahler, M., Pine, F., & Bergman, A. (1975) *The Psychological Birth of the Human Infant*. New York: Basic Books.
Maslow, A. (1968) *Toward a Psychology of Being*. New York: Van Nostrand Reinhold.
Masterson, J.F. (1981) *The Narcissistic and Borderline Disorders*. New York: Brunner/Mazel.
Mitchell, S.A. & Black, M. (1995) *Freud and Beyond*, New York: Basic Books.
Siegel, D.J. (2007) *The Mindful Brain*. New York: Norton.
Smith, J.R. (1986) Margaret S. Mahler, MD: Original thinker, exceptional woman. In Dickstein, L.J. & Nadelson, C.C. (eds) *Women Physicians in Leadership Roles*. Washington, DC: American Psychiatric Press.
Solnit, A. (1986) Anna Freud: Bold investigator and model builder. In Dickstein, L.J. & Nadelson, C.C. (eds) *Women Physicians in Leadership Roles*. Washington, DC: American Psychiatric Press.
Spitz, R. (1946a) Hospitalism: A follow-up report. *Psychoanalytic Study of the Child*, 2: 113–117.
Spitz, R. (1946b) Anaclitic depression. *Psychoanalytic Study of the Child*, 2: 313–342.
Spitz, R. (1965) *The First Year of Life*. New York: International Universities Press.
Young-Bruehl, E. (1988) *Anna Freud: A Biography*. New York: Norton.

5

THE MIDDLE SCHOOL

With good enough mothering, we evolve from ruthless to "ruth"

In the late 1940s, the British psychoanalytical society split into three, each section claiming loyalty to Freud. Melanie Klein and Anna Freud had their very separate and at times hostile camps separated in both theory and how to train future analysts. Anna Freud's position was that the goal of analysis was to enlarge and enrich the ego enabling it to manage the id; Klein's was less ambitious theorizing that the best that can be done is lower anxiety (Grosskurth, 1986; Young-Bruehl, 1988). At the time, everyone had to choose which side to be on or join the so-called middle group. Perhaps it is to the credit of these divided colleagues that they were and are able to remain under one umbrella and sometimes continue their conversations. Nevertheless, their differences were and are profound.

It is with the clinical and theoretical contributions of this British middle school that our understanding of particular struggles of the mind opens up even more dramatically. These practitioners focused on deeply debilitating invisible issues, such as shame, anxiety, depression, and inner deadness. All were influenced directly by both Klein and Anna Freud and all are part of the early object-relations school of thought. Nevertheless, their stance is so different that for me they deserve a legacy line all their own. These contributors possessed an uncanny ability to empathize with their suffering patients—perhaps because they themselves had suffered in similar ways. Although all were classical analysts, they were much less interested in being "objective" when they were with their patients. Instead, they sought some form of "relating to" and "being with" the patient. It is here that psychoanalytic discourse begins to change from strictly objective to somewhat subjective. All else stayed the same: the couch, the lack of eye contact, seeing people many times a week, etc. The most influential and prolific of these middle school contributors was D.W. Winnicott, but I will present each of them chronologically.

RONALD FAIRBAIRN

A native of Scotland, Ronald Fairbairn (1889–1964) first studied moral philosophy. After serving in World War I, he trained as a doctor, with interests in psychology, adolescence, and "war neurosis." While in medical school, he read Freud in the original, underwent an analysis and, as was the practice of that time, started practicing as a psychoanalyst in 1925 with no further training. By 1938, he was a highly regarded member of the British Psychoanalytical Society. Fairbairn was known for his independent thinking. He lived his entire life in Edinburgh, which may have contributed to his singularity. London, the center of psychoanalysis and psychoanalytic controversies and pressures, was a difficult journey by train, not easily undertaken (Gomez, 1997).

War neurosis

The consequences of trauma, such as war, rape, and childhood abuse, are now universally consolidated under the category of post-traumatic stress disorder, or PTSD (Herman, 1992). Sadly, during the two Great Wars, when a man returned from combat with tremendous upset and an inability to resume normal life, he was stigmatized as having a "war neurosis." Britain had large facilities dedicated to helping these shattered soldiers return to normal life, recognizing their need for some help and provision (Fairbairn, 1943, 1952).

Our need for others

Fairbairn made seminal contributions to the foundation of object relations as a distinct psychological theory. In 1941, he proposed that *people are the objects of drives*, thus forsaking the Freudian perspective that the pleasure of discharge is the goal of a drive (Gomez, 1997). This was a huge change in thinking, extremely controversial, and for the most part ignored at the time. For Klein, "object" referred to an internal event, built into our being and disconnected from external experience. For Fairbairn, objects were real, separate people in the external environment that the infant needed for its survival. By reformulating Freud's drive theory, Fairbairn changed the focus of both theory and practice in dramatic ways. His model is much more interpersonal than biological. Moreover, he was the first to write about the primacy of the real mother–child relationship to the developing self. It is impossible to overstate the significance of this shift of focus for the analytic project from exclusive concern with the inner life of phantasy to balancing those concerns with the necessary relationships with other real persons (Fairbairn, 1943, 1952; Gomez, 1997).

For Freud and Klein, the given or natural inner world is composed of our personal creations, either from primary process thinking (Freud) or the two fundamental positions (Klein). Fairbairn, on the other hand, was committed to understanding the lived experience of his patients, what they actually endured, most especially when they were very young. He contended the ego or self is whole at birth, and lived experience creates unavoidable conflicts. Of course, different people will make different things out of the same experience; every person will be deeply affected by his or her personal experience, shaped by family contact, and distorted by painful events, such as war or child abuse.

Fairbairn (1952) argued that, from the beginning of life, there is a predetermined need to seek out real and separate others. This need for others is inborn and primary. When relating to others, the child experiences both bad and good moments, thus creating his mind, shaping his personal way of thinking, and constructing his way of being in the world. All this is totally bound to the baby's lived experiences with real others. Fairbairn's theory of early development and psychopathology is based on actual and concrete environmental success and failure. The more the environment fails the baby, the more fixated or frozen in the past the developing self becomes. Fairbairn contended that we always become somewhat like our parents, most particularly in those ways in which they have failed us. This wounding remains our lifelong connection to them. These fixated or frozen aspects of ourselves are difficult to relinquish, for letting go of them threatens our connections to these first love objects, who were or should have been the source of safety and survival. We internalize our first relationships, both positive and negative, creating a sense of self that is subtly discontinuous and, at the same time, ongoing. Fairbairn was particularly interested in real contact with his patients and noted that when they could not make contact with him they could not effectively relate to their significant others (Klein, J., 1987).

Dynamic structures

Fairbairn maintained, like Freud and Klein, that at the beginning of life the baby could not distinguish between self and other, nor from where any felt distress originates. The baby's needs are mysterious forces emerging out of nowhere and being satisfied or not. Fairbairn's first dynamic structures are formulated from his belief in this pre-personal oneness of mother-and-baby-are-one. For him, at birth the baby is whole and relates to a necessary other hopefully feeling loved and that his love is received in turn.

Fairbairn hypothesizes three early universal object relationships: exciting or libidinal (keeping to Freud's language), anti-libidinal, and one shorn of powerful feelings altogether (Fairbairn, 1943, 1952). When the aroused baby must wait too long for satisfaction, the baby creates the tantalizing phantasy that there is an object, an other, that is wonderful but not fully present. This is the frustrating mother, who Fairbairn named the "exciting object." I find it easier to imagine what he is thinking about by calling it the "frustrating exciting object." While internally enthralled with the frustrating exciting object, the babe creates a corresponding partial self, which Fairbairn named the "libidinal ego." These two sides of the relationship fuel and define each other and cannot be considered as existing without each other. Frustrating exciting object ↔ libidinal ego.

At the same time, within this same infant, another pair of relationships is developing with a darker tone. When the mother does not sufficiently provide for the baby, he experiences a "rejecting object," creating his personal internal saboteur, or sadistic superego. This pair is anti-pleasure and anti-life. Rejecting object ↔ sadistic superego. Experiencing the first pair reawakens need, while the second creates rage and hostility and leads to despair and hopelessness. Everyone has both pairs; they are both normal and if terribly out of balance, the source of psychopathology.

Together these pairs drain energy from the original whole self, creating what Fairbairn called the "central ego." This structure is much less capable of experiencing the emotional aspects of aliveness; it is invested in management. It does the remembering, the perceiving, the comparing and planning. The central ego exists at the boundary of the self and others and its relational companion in the external world is the ideal object. Central ego ↔ ideal object. This pair is conscious—if I am good you will love me and take care of me—while the other two pairs are repressed in Fairbairn's model. Like the other dynamic pairs, the central ego ↔ ideal object are universal and problematical (Gomez, 1997).

Schizoid factors

As previously noted, Fairbairn's most famous statement is that the human baby is object-seeking, not discharge-seeking. A second important concept emerged from his observation that, when needs are not met, the child may turn deeply inward to an unwholesome depth, depending on his own fantasy life to meet all of his needs. This preoccupation with inner fantasy along with an attitude of omnipotence and detachment constitutes what Fairbairn calls "schizoid factors." These are foundational in all of us and problematic to many. Fairbairn proposed that the original cause of schizoid factors is separation anxiety. This happens when a young child cannot bear prolonged absence from his mother. When no one is there, the baby must attend to himself in a precocious manner. To a baby, separation anxiety equals death (Fairbairn, 1943, 1952).

Fairbairn also wrote extensively and elaborately on the phenomenon of "splitting," wherein the child conceives of a good parent and a bad parent and is unable to create a healthy, ambivalent whole parent. At the same time, there is a good self and a bad self paired with these structures. Splitting is a result of environmental failure, not only a failure of imagination. Due to lack of sufficient care, the baby has been unable to weave positive and negative experiences into a unifying notion of a complex other (Klein, J., 1987). When treating suffering individuals, Fairbairn was clear that to heal, insight alone is not enough. It will not bring change. The recovering patient must experience that the new is possible. He needs to concretely experience others with whom he can form a real, caring relationship. It is lived emotional experience that brings change. Mental understanding is necessary but not sufficient (Fairbairn, 1943, 1952; Mitchell & Black, 1995).

"Don" is a writer, in his forties, never married, and always longing for a relationship. He shares little about his childhood. He tells me his parents were just fine, if a little distant and preoccupied with making a living. When we sit together, Don is very quiet, in a way that is quite different from Jess. When Jess is quiet, I sense her inner activity. We are both in reverie. I am confident that if I wait, Jess will find her words and her energy and feelings will emerge. I do not have that same experience with Don. The quiet is hard on both of us. He explicitly asks that I break the quiet, saying that he cannot. He does not know what to say, has no idea what is important, or what he might like to explore. Thanks to an internet dating service, Dan is currently seeing someone and hopes that this matures into a relationship. At the same time, he is passive, unable to create his own next steps. As we sit together, Don can articulate questions he would like to ask the woman he is seeing. When they are together, he remains frozen and never finds the right time. When we are quiet together and I ask what goes on inside, his first answer is always "Nothing." His face is very held, so it is hard for me to guess what feelings move through him. I ask about any fantasies regarding this relationship and its future. With a nervous laugh, he answers: "We need to spend more time together; I don't really think about it in that way. I just know I would be happier if I had a relationship."

Don sits with me in great stillness; his emotions do not move; his fantasies are not allowed to come to consciousness. He goes blank in my presence. It is as if in the waiting for connection, Don has given up, gone numb or dead. I ask him what it is like to come to therapy, to be with me. Once again, his response is bland: It is fine. Do you look forward to coming? "Sorta. It is the only time I try to think about me and not the book I am writing." Don knows both himself and others to be complex and contradictory. I deeply appreciate Fairbairn's insights concerning what he called schizoid phenomena, as they give me some guidance as to what questions to ask that might stimulate connection. I am poignantly aware of how important it is to stay vivid myself and to lean into the situation by reflecting his feelings as I discern them and steadfastly refusing to enact his numbness and deadness by becoming distant and passive myself.

Even though he lived and worked in relative isolation in Scotland, Fairbairn was concerned about psychoanalysis as a whole and wished it to be an embedded part of contemporary culture. He wanted its theories to be consistent, and for clinical practice to be tied rigorously and directly to those theories. Of course, he did not get that professional desire fulfilled; rather he lived through the upsetting and open hostilities between Anna Freud and Klein with no resolution whatsoever.

MICHAEL BALINT

Michael Balint (1896–1970) was born Mihály Maurice Bergsmann in Budapest, Hungary. Estranged from his father, he eventually changed both his religion and his name. Balint sustained a serious wound while serving in World War I, which allowed him to return to medical school where he avidly read Freud. Due to his experiences of both war and medical school, his first passion was psychosomatics. He had two two-year analyses, one with the then ostracized Ferenczi, neither very satisfactory by his own accounts (Gomez, 1997). Nevertheless, by the mid-1920s, as he was intrigued by the theory and possibilities of the method, he presented himself as an analyst. He practiced in Budapest until war again intruded upon his life, then moved to England in 1939. There, he produced his most significant contributions, writing exclusively in English. He found a natural home in the British psychoanalytic world of the 1940s. Already interested in the mother–infant relationship before his forced move, Balint found a vibrant context for these interests in the early childhood theories posited by both Klein and Anna Freud.

The basic fault

For me, Balint's most important psychoanalytic contribution is his understanding of those early years. His is a very different development model from those mentioned so far. First, he proposed what he called the "area of creation" (somewhat like Mahler's autistic stage), where the baby is presumed to be self-contained and simply waiting for its needs to be met. There are no external objects/others whatsoever in this stage of development. This is followed by the first two-person relationship, comprising baby and mother. He called this the area of the "basic fault." The nature and quality of this first two-person relationship sets the stage for everything that follows (Balint, 1968, 1979; Klein, J., 1987) If this goes well, then the "normal" conflicts of the later three-personal relationship of mother, father, and child—Freud's Oedipal conflict—will emerge. This implies that the unfolding Oedipal stage of development is not guaranteed. Instead, it depends on the success of the much earlier mother–baby dyad.

Primary love

Balint called that first object relationship between infant and mother "primary love," and he wrote about the effects of this love in his own life and the lives of his patients. This self-disclosure was unusual in the psychoanalytic community. To write about himself so personally and to use the word "love" as a key concept in this developmental theory were both previously unacceptable in the science of psychoanalysis. Balint wrote that, in a good environment, the infant experiences his specific other as totally available. This available other is more like a substance to be used than a separate person. His felicitous phrase "harmonious interpenetrating mix-up" captures his intended meaning completely (Balint, 1968, 1979). Like the relationship of fish to water or humans to air, the relationship is effortless; things simply "are." Within this loving situation, the baby is not "done to" but rather loved and cared for; his needs are met before they become painful demands. Most of the time, the mother enjoys caring for her baby. Within this generous context, the baby enjoys and thrives in the harmonious mix-up, without awareness of his needs because they are met. He does not experience himself as prematurely separate. This baby lives in a healthy illusion of oneness and develops his potential because of the blessing of harmonious interdependence (Gomez, 1997).

Breaking the illusion of oneness

In order for the baby to discover that others have a separate existence, this harmonious interdependence must be interrupted. This happens within the first year of life, triggering the individuation process. Balint wrote that initially there are two possible and diametrically opposed unconscious reactions to this crucial discovery that others are not in total alignment. In one phantasy, others are kind and useful, and merger with them is desirable. In the other phantasy, others are deemed as not necessary or even nonexistent. In the latter phantasy of no others, the baby experiences no obstacles to personal will and power (Klein, J., 1987).

In the instance of the first phantasy type, the developing child turns to others as saviors and creates strong interpersonal relationships. The unconscious cost is that of mistrusting unique and personal inner needs, ideas, and creations—deferring to others in order to keep the connection at all costs. In some cases, the personal sense of self is that of "less than" or unworthy. The connection is more important than the personal call of individuation and being whole.

Within the phantasy of the second type, others are unconsciously experienced as either dangerous or irrelevant, to be avoided or used as needed. People of this group cultivate independence, skills, and prioritize looking after themselves. They resist needing others, especially a particular other. They trust themselves and their values and tend to act as if their way of being in the world is the only or best way.

Jess is a good example of the first type. She seeks to stay close to her husband and her mother and finds it very difficult to express her own needs, especially when they conflict with the needs of her special others. Don is a good example of the second. He highly values his independence and his freedom. He chooses his projects carefully and lives precisely where and how he wants to live. Don is successful in a public sense and very lonely at the personal level.

Within Balint's model, both of these types have limits and strengths. As unconscious reactions to the individuation journey, each can be the foundation for unintegrated ambivalence toward both others and self. We can be too dependent and needy, or alternatively too separate, superior, and condescending. He wrote that when we bring to consciousness our personal, previously unconscious reactions to others, those who are overly dependent can create true intimacy while maintaining a separate sense of self; those who love space and separateness can follow their call for curiosity and explorations and, at the same time, learn to trust another.

For me, Balint's ideas change the stance of the analyst in very important ways (Balint, 1965). The classical Freudian, including most of the Kleinians and ego psychologists, is a traditional father figure—a good, distant authority, offering interpretations and clear boundaries. Balint (like Fairbairn) pictured the good analyst more as a benign mother figure—able and willing to be used to enter the split world of the basic fault, where the growth process can reignite and then develop. This maternal framing supports the inclusion of the word "love" in the analytic conversation. As indicated previously, this was a dramatic addition to the lexicon.

When I sit with Mary I am acutely aware of Balint's basic fault. This is the world in which Mary lives. She plunges into her "bad." Her envy, rage, and despair can consume her entire way of being. Mary frequently questions whether staying alive is worth all the pain. Yet, abandoning her autistic son would be unthinkable. Mary questions my capacity to empathize, to care for her. She searches my face for a trace of disgust, listens intently to my tone for a trace of dismissiveness— looking for proof that I, like her mother, find her despicable. Mary needs understanding but that will not be enough. She needs a lived experience of my emotional involvement, my care and concern, and also my outrage at how she was treated as a child.

According to Balint, when the patient needs to explore the level of the basic fault, they must be allowed to "regress to a state of dependency." Only through appropriate regression can a "new beginning" be ignited (Balint, 1968, 1979). Balint urged working slowly with these cases. There must be no insistence, interpretations, or challenging confrontations. Projections and even acting out are to be expected and tolerated. He also recognized that the need to cling, to regress and depend, was not always a return to primary love; rather, it also could indicate a response to trauma, to the fear of being abandoned. For Balint, this is the return to the basic fault, the area of early relational trauma in order to come into a new beginning

Benign versus malignant regression

Balint gave us the very important distinction between benign and malignant regression. Within benign regression during a long-term therapy, basic trust can be (re)created and the patient's demands for gratification can be managed at a moderate level. The analyst can recognize the need presented and help the patient find the best solution (perhaps by holding his hand) to the very real need. Malignant regression feels very different. Here, the patient becomes intensely demanding. Often, if one set of needs is met, demands then escalate. Within a malignant regression, the analyst is at risk of becoming controlled by the demands of the patient, creating intense frustration without any resolution. Balint highly valued being an unobtrusive therapist, not a savior or a sage (Balint, 1968, 1979).

In addition to his work in psychoanalysis, Balint was very interested in the benefits of supportive professional groups. In 1950, he initiated supportive groups for general practitioners in England, a reflection of groups he had created in Hungary 25 years earlier. Another of his projects was the doctor-patient relationship for primary-care physicians. His book *The Doctor, His Patient and the Illness* (1957) provided the foundation for the establishment of the Balint Society and the Balint Groups, which continue to this day. For legal reasons, Balint retired at age 65. This freed him to travel, to focus on his interest in these professional groups, and overall to disseminate his ideas (Gomez, 1997).

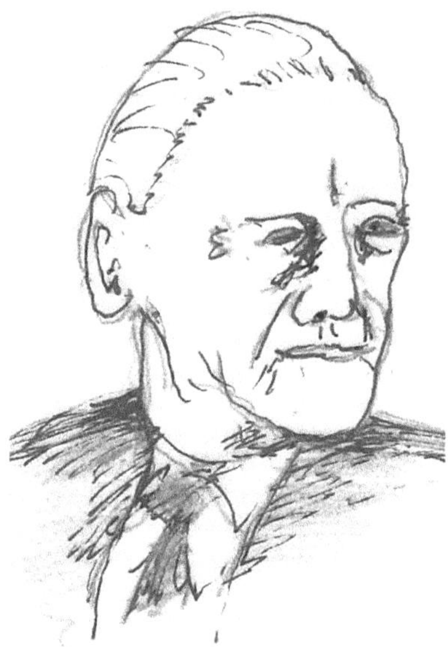

Donald Winnicott

DONALD WINNICOTT

Unlike so many of his important colleagues, Donald Winnicott (1896–1971) was British through and through. Although he had not completed medical school, he served as a medical officer in World War I. During World War II, he was a consulting psychiatrist to the evacuee program. Winnicott trained first as a pediatrician and practiced pediatrics throughout his life. During his psychoanalytic training in the 1920s, he undertook two analyses—one of which spanned 10 years—and also studied with Klein (Rodman, 2003).

Winnicott is best explored through the many new concepts he introduced into the analytic conversation. It is important to acknowledge how radical they were for the time and how important they remain today. In comparison to his contemporaries his writing style is casual, usually without references; nor is it linear, rather it is more impressionistic, circling the experience and ideas he is discussing.

True and false self

One of Winnicott's boldest theoretical leaps was to propose the existence of a "true self," an internal source of wholeness and goodness that is always present though often hidden. We create defenses, "false selves," to protect this true self. I love both of these concepts—that we have a source of knowing what is right and good for us and that when we are not safe and cannot trust, we will create protection for that same vulnerability. When safety is insured, the true self will emerge (Winnicott, 1960a). Winnicott provides yet another lens to view the individuation journey. In his later writing, he suggests that each analyst must find his unique way of welcoming the unconscious fragments of self, rather than confronting an unconscious full of negativity or resistance. Waiting for the unfolding, rather than pushing by interpretation was his intent (Winnicott, 1968).

With every one of the patients I have mentioned, in this way of thinking there is a true self looking for its own best way to find expression. When Don "goes dead," when Mary hates herself and others, when Charlie enumerates his net worth one more time, I trust that these are their best expressions of the moment, even though I might personally find these repetitive expressions frustrating. Don needs an enlivening other who is attuned to the presence of what Winnicott called his "spontaneous gestures of emotional creativity." Mary needs compassion and understanding that her hate is a valid protest—pointing to unmet needs beneath—and this protest can be softened and humanized. Charlie needs hope that there is more to him than his net worth. Using the concept of a true self engaged on its own individuation journey frames these different systems and helps me stay centered and in dialogue with a deeper part of each of these clients who lives primarily in his or her defenses.

Life at the beginning

Winnicott disagreed with Klein and Fairbairn over the primacy of negative emotions. His experience was that the positive, creative potential for life was also present from the beginning. He argued that Klein's primary emotions of hate and envy require "intention," and that, at the beginning of life, there is no conscious intention. There is only the need for contact and survival (Winnicott, 1963a). He proposed that when the baby is in a good environment, they live in a comfortable, unintegrated stream, which he termed "going-on-being." This is a big contrast to Klein's terrified infant. Winnicott did acknowledge that infants are ruthless, and that getting their needs met is a matter of life and death—very much an id phenomenon.

As Klein was his mentor, it is logical that, first, he wanted to ground Kleinian theory in observable reality. However, over time, as he worked both with infants, as a pediatrician, and with adults and children, as a psychiatrist, he slowly went his own way. For him, this ruthlessness has little to do with the phantasies of Kleinian drive language; instead, it is a necessary developmental stage that ensures survival before the awareness of real others. With that developing awareness comes "ruth." Ruth is that essential aliveness which comes from the bodily lust of nursing plus the developing capacity for concern for that real, separate other (Winnicott, 1963b).

As he observed children and mothers directly, he saw the tremendous impact that others have on the developing child. At the same time, Winnicott always supported the classical one-person position of psychoanalysis, that our life is largely of our own making and that we repeat what we have experienced. He strongly believed that, in analysis, it is best to focus on the wish, the fantasy, and personal character as revealed in his consulting room, rather than what others have done to us (Mitchell & Black, 1995).

From his observations came one of his most famous statements: There is no such thing as a baby, there is only a mother–baby dyad (Winnicott, 1960b) His phrase "primary maternal preoccupation" refers to the new mother's all-encompassing, exclusive focus on the newborn for its first months of life (Winnicott, 1956). This invites the baby's true self to emerge. In the right context, the ruthless infant develops ruth, which includes the ability to care for others. Over time, the initial ruthlessness will develop into "capacity for concern."

The notion of the "good enough mother" is another Winnicott gem. She is not the split Kleinian good mother; she is much more than that (Abram, 1996). She is not perfect, but she is attuned and attentive. She allows her particular baby to "find himself" in and through her care. During those first months of life, the good enough mother presents the baby with the illusion that he is omnipotent, that he can have what he wants whenever he wants it. She encourages him to hold the illusion that he creates the breast or bottle that feeds him when he is hungry. She is a safe and secure "holding environment." She is the baby's first mirror—giving him through her face his agency, his creativity, his emotional reality, not reflecting back her separateness, her mood, or concerns (Winnicott, 1964; 1967). For the baby to become real to itself, to connect with and begin to live from his true self, Winnicott believed that the maternal environment must do all of the adapting at the very beginning. A baby can be fed without love, but impersonal management will not call forth a new, autonomous human being.

The two mothers

Winnicott found many parallels between the early mother–baby relationship and psychoanalysis. He was conscious of the importance of good mothering, both for the developing infant and for society as a whole. He used his insights around the theme of the good enough mother to inform his position as an analyst and to educate the mothers of Great Britain on his radio broadcasts for parents (Winnicott, 1988). He hypothesized that, in the beginning, the infant experiences the mother in two very different ways. She is at the same time the "environmental mother" and also the "object mother." The environmental mother is a "substance to be used," much as Balint suggested. The object mother is a true other, who will slowly help her child to relinquish the idea that the entire world revolves around him. The analyst, too, holds both of these positions in the mind of the patient. Sometimes, the analyst will create the environment necessary to meet the patient's needs to be mirrored and understood. Sometimes, the analyst will be an objective other, offering an interpretation or a different point of view, while still keeping the other in mind (Winnicott, 1963b).

Transitional objects

As a pediatrician, Winnicott noticed that many children had special soft toys or bits of blankets that they treasured. These items gave the child a sense of security. He proposed that this special item somehow stands in for the mother and holds some of her power of safety and protection. He named such items "transitional objects." The transitional object is neither subjectively created and controlled nor discovered and separate. It is both; it is a wonderful paradox. It is important that the parents do not challenge the child's connection with their transitional object. Wise parents know that at some point in the future the object will lose its significance. But meanwhile, it must not be washed—as that can change its smell and, therefore, its value—and it must not disappear—as that would be a traumatic loss (Winnicott, 1951).

Transitional space

Slowly, over the baby's first year of life, objective reality comes to co-exist with subjective reality. Hopefully, the baby lives in the experience that their spontaneity is real and important. Between objective reality and subjective reality lies transitional space or potential space. Between creating and finding is that same wonderful paradoxical dimension of living. Like the transitional object, transitional space is both objective and subjective, real and imagined. This domain is terribly important. It is the area where play and creativity happen, and, for Winnicott, this also is the space of good psychotherapy. He was ever concerned with the quality of subjective experience, with its capacity to infuse life with meaning. The baby and the patient both need that creative space to find themselves and connect to their spontaneous gestures permitting change and growth. Over time, he viewed this as a protected realm, within which the true self, the creative self, could quicken and play, eventually creating art and culture (Winnicott, 1951).

Collecting impingements

When the needs of the environment and the needs of the child are at odds, the child is "impinged" upon. On the one hand, he could feel ignored, as if he and his needs don't matter. Alternatively, he might be forced into "compliance" with the outer authority. Wherever and whenever a child experiences an impingement, they will then unconsciously register that this is the nature of the world (Winnicott, 1960b). Then they will unconsciously recreate this arrangement over and over again. This is the source of the split between the spontaneous wellsprings of desire and meaning (true self) and the compliant self (false self). If there is a "sin" in Winnicott's lexicon, it is compliance. For Winnicott, it is immoral to force anyone to comply at the expense of their personal way of life. Being required to comply, to grow up, and to fit in, destroys the uniqueness of each individual. Only in the safety of spontaneity can the true self reveal itself and the individual find their own creative way in the world. Winnicott wrote that, as therapists, our purpose is not to pursue research on patients as objects, nor to cure; rather, it is to create some meaningful interaction along with some capacity to play, opening the possibility for further self-discovery (Winnicott, 1971; Davis & Wallbridge, 1981; Mitchell & Black, 1995).

> *Don has lost his spontaneity, his basic aliveness. His bland presentation of both his history and his emotional needs suggests that his spontaneity was not mirrored or valued in his earliest years. As a result, he has lost connection with his emotional wellsprings. He knows something is missing in his life, but he has neither words nor a felt sense of what it might be.*

Play

Winnicott highly valued what he called "play" and wrote about it over and over. Children must play spontaneously in order to express their true self. Psychotherapy is conducted in the overlapping of two areas of play, one of the therapist, the other of the patient. For him, play is the opposite of the premature development of an organized self or personality. Play allows a truly integrated self to emerge in its own time, without compliance, and happy just to "be." Play is a way of discovering and knowing oneself, trusting one's impulses, free of anxiety or premature organization. He proposed that it is only during play that the individual can be fully creative and discover his whole self: his personality—conscious and unconscious, integrated and non-integrated (Winnicott, 1971).

Therapy

Winnicott used case examples from both children and adults in many if not most of his writings. We learn even more about his attitude and style from his 1947 paper, "Hate in the counter-transference." Winnicott did not believe in innate Kleinian hate. But he did believe that the mother hates her baby before the baby hates its mother. He suggested that without the emotional freedom to hate, there cannot be love. The capacity to hate is a developmental achievement, and he encouraged each analyst to know his own capacity to hate, including hating his patients at certain moments. He wrote that the time limit of each session is an expression of that hate. He devised the ideas of "objective love" and "objective hate" to acknowledge that there are aspects of patients that deserve our hate, and that this hate must be "stored" and sorted and eventually offered as an interpretation at the right time.

For Winnicott, the analyst must put his own subjectivity on hold, just like the good enough mother. He offered refuge to his patients. He contended that content and interpretation were less important than the crucial experience of the self in relation to the other. Only that would enable the patient to rediscover his own capacity to imagine and create, feel real and meaningful. This is, by necessity, an emotional relationship where both individuals are internally alive to themselves and to each other.

We know even more about his approach thanks to Margaret Little and Harry Guntrip (discussed later), both of whom were analyzed by him and wrote about their experiences. Winnicott always claimed to work in the classical manner, acknowledging his allegiance to Freud, even though it is very doubtful that Freud himself worked in the very astringent, neutral manner of the stereotype. The report by Little, also a doctor and analyst, of her work with him is anything but neutral or astringent. During many intense periods, she saw him seven days a week and, if ill, he came to her. During those periods, he held her hands constantly even though they both knew it was physically uncomfortable for him. He also held her head when she needed. Because she needed a long period of quiet before speaking, he extended their time together without raising her fee. He insisted that she be safe in hospital while he was away on vacation for fear of suicide. When, in a fury, she broke things precious to him, he let her know but did not punish her. Her report is certainly one of deep care, even love (Little, 1977).

He expected long-term therapy to take time and wrote about how these long-term, intense treatments were affecting him. He acknowledged that the immaturity and dependence of certain patients had an impact on his well-being, and he cautioned that the analyst must always be aware of that impact. He acknowledged his own humanity and limitations. He wrote eloquently on how difficult, challenging, and personally painful an analysis can be (Winnicott, 1954; Little 1977).

Winnicott acknowledged that therapists need their own self-care system and have to indirectly communicate to their patients that they themselves do not need to be taken care of (by the patient). Importantly, therapists must stay separate, keeping an independent reality from the various anxieties of the patient. Winnicott called this "survival," without wounding the other or getting ahead of the other's developmental capabilities. He compared it to the mother's survival of the infant's ruthless needs and rages. Therapists and mothers need to survive and not retaliate. This does not mean there is not an impact but, rather, that the impact is managed by the adult aspect of the therapist's self (Winnicott, 1968).

I think of Winnicott as an optimist in the sense of having faith in each of his patients that they could find their way with a reflecting, mirroring other.

He believed that a foundational trust was created by the baby and the good enough mother and that foundational trust needed to be created or re-created within the analytic relationship.

Winnicott used the word "trust" developmentally. He wrote that trust is the building up of confidence based on experience, in the time of maximum dependence, before the enjoyment and employment of separation and of independence. He trusted the goodwill of the patient. He saw symptoms, dreams, and regressions as expressions of the verbally incommunicable. These actions and fantasies speak the unspeakable. If the analyst can trust the patient, himself, and the work and play of psychoanalysis, the traumatically frozen incident or primary relationship, over time, will thaw, words will be found, understanding and meaning created (Winnicott,1954).

The composite clients I have introduced you to here challenge me in many ways. Can I stay alive in the presence of Don's lack of feelings? Can I manage my exasperation without undue anger or retaliation when Jack doesn't respond to my emails? When Mary demands that I prove to her that she is not horrible, how do I stay authentic? Winnicott's beautiful idea of building trust is a cornerstone for long-term work; trust in the relationship, trust in the other, and trust in the self. All over time.

Even though Winnicott wrote extensively about the interactions between patient and analyst, his was still a one-person model of healing and change. He knew how important the relationship was (Phillips, 1988) and, yet, at the same time, his focus was on the drives and developmental steps within each patient. He clearly modified the classical stance of neutrality when the situation demanded it and believed in being emotionally alive and present as the healing context, with interpretation only second. Winnicott, unlike Balint, never talked of love when referring to his patients, but as we read Little (1977) the word must certainly apply.

Fear of breakdown

My patient Jack experiences himself as "falling apart" and worries that he will fall beyond hope of return. Winnicott gives me wise counsel: Clinical fear of breakdown, he writes, is the fear of a breakdown that has already been experienced (Winnicott, 1963c; Little, 1977). Jack had such a tumultuous early beginning. He experienced unthinkable anxieties again and again. Our job now is to acknowledge that what he is experiencing in the present is colored by his past. However, in the present, and in the presence of a connected other, he can experience intensely painful emotional experiences and come out on the other side. This was not possible in his early years of life.

HARRY GUNTRIP

Like Fairbairn and Winnicott, Harry Guntrip (1901–1975) was British. He first became a Protestant minister, later a psychologist, and then a psychoanalyst with no formal training beyond first an analysis with Fairbairn and later one with Winnicott. He was deeply introspective, keeping detailed written records of his dreams and his experiences in analysis. Guntrip's personal trauma stemmed from the death of his younger brother, when Guntrip was around 3 years old. He carried this memory all his life and believed that it was the source of his own inner deadness, depressions, mysterious illnesses, and despair—his own "schizoid phenomena." He deeply hoped that the second analysis, the one with Winnicott, would allow him to regress into the childhood state, and memories of his personal trauma finally bring some healing. Indeed, his whole personality expanded and vitalized due to that experience (Hazell, 1996). He took extensive notes during his analyses and from those notes we can gather both how Winnicott and Fairbairn worked and the interpretations they offered.

Like Fairbairn and Balint, Guntrip was deeply interested in schizoid phenomena, the problem of being unable to maintain a sense of internal ongoingness around others without self fragmentation. He advanced the thinking of the object-relations school by writing personally and thoughtfully about his experiences with these withdrawn, often isolated patients. In the last chapter of *Psychoanalytic Theory, Therapy, and the Self* (1971), Guntrip insists that technique will not cure these early traumas; rather, they need a "real" relationship with a "real other." This was very different from the neutral interpretative stance advocated by most of his peers at the time. Guntrip and Balint both directly encouraged therapists and analysts to risk really caring for the people who entered their offices. They believed that analysis is more than a job, it is a calling, and the analyst must live in his own spontaneous being to follow that calling.

Guntrip (1969) wrote about other analysts' ideas and then added his own important contributions. For example, when writing about Fairbairn's developmental model of dependence, independence, and interdependence, he added the concept of "pre-moral" as part of those early stages of life. I find this a very useful clinical formulation when struggling with a patient's felt need to use, manipulate, even harm others with total justification. A developmental arrest is easier to sit with and explore than a moral failure.

He wrote extensively about the need for analysis to focus on the earliest stages of life, the pre-Oedipal years. His writing is warm, and he uses the word "love" extensively, talking about the human need for love, how love is frozen when the infant is not properly mirrored and cared for, the various distortions that love can take, and how important the love is between therapist and patient. The first year of life, when the baby is sorting out "me" and "you" and "us," is crucial in his view. Loving care—referred to as the "proper environment"—is critical for these internal structures to form. We all need a sense of us, a merger with an other at the beginning, in order to bear the ordinary distresses of life. Without the possibility of safe others, life becomes too difficult. Without a sense of a good us, the me never becomes strong enough to exist without the terrors of fragmenting. For Guntrip, the poor environment imprints a very difficult unconscious inner world, where needs are stimulated and tantalized but never given satisfaction. He believed that all people have an irreducible need for love, and if that love was not forthcoming at the beginning of life, we are left in a permanently painful state. His model of the self involved deficit and trauma from early years, not inner drives and conflicts (Klein, J., 1987).

Early inner states

Guntrip wrote that in his experience there were two possible reactions when infants do not receive their needed love: "love made angry" and "love made hungry." Love made angry corresponds to depressive anxieties and attempts to force love from the other. Of course, this then engenders fear that the other will be angry in return and leave. Alternatively, it can create guilt at hurting or upsetting the other. In an adult, all of these reactions can generate a kind of depression and depletion of internal resources. With enough agency or ego strength, this type of adult may leave to look for someone else to connect with and to love.

Love made hungry, corresponding with schizoid anxieties, describes the sense of becoming more and more needy, and desperately craving contact with the loved one. This cycle unfolds into the fear that the individual's love is too much and will overwhelm—or even psychologically destroy—the beloved, resulting in abandonment. The depression that follows this sequence results in a fierce distancing from the loved one. This kind of dismissive depression forecloses the possibilities of second chances. Loving becomes too dangerous, and aloneness is the only possibility (Klein, J., 1987).

Mary is an excellent example of what happens as a consequence of a lack of love in early life, as described by Guntrip. With her husband, she alternates between love made angry and love made hungry. In the Kleinian model, I, the therapist, must bring into awareness her envy and greed, relate these painful feelings to her past, and highlight the impossibility of satiation in the present. Informed by the work of Winnicott and Guntrip, I can empathize with Mary's longing for love and understand her distorted ways of attempting to extract it from her current family. I can acknowledge that her longing is real and should have been met in her earliest years, and I can confirm that there is nothing fundamentally wrong with her longing or her needs. Then, together, we can explore how her style of attempting to get the love and connection she craves needs refining in order to achieve what she both longs for and has a right to. Can I help Mary separate the genuine need from the dysfunctional action?

Rejecting her need leaves Mary full of self-hate. We must sit together with the truth and the force of her need. I help her hold and contain her angry feelings of deprivation, so she can create a different perspective for both herself and her situation. Can we enter the grief of what should have been and cannot be?

Accepting her grief and her needs allows some inner space and some self-acceptance.

Guntrip utilized Fairbairn's three theoretical object relationships with an important addition that he called the regressed ego. This fragment of self withdraws to an imaginary womb, contained but without others completely (Gomez, 1997). This regressed ego has given up and needs no one. He was poignantly empathic to the dilemma of those who both dread and crave relationship. For people caught in this dilemma, relationships present a terrifying choice: To be loved is to be swallowed up and lost; alternatively, to love is to take over the other person and consume their identity. There is no capacity for an "us" or "we" identity. There are only the devastating extremes of separateness or merger (Klein, J., 1987). In his experience, in the first year of life, "me and not me," along with "you" and "us" are experienced in Balint's "interpenetrating mix-up." With good enough care, the different structures of the self consolidate: There is a me, a you, and sometimes an us. When care is inadequate, these structures may fail to form, creating an adult like Mary, full of psychic distress and stretched between two unacceptable alternatives: dreadful aloneness or psychic merger and disappearance.

According to Guntrip, this is where good psychotherapy might intervene. Only by finding someone outside of themselves who can care for them, understand them, and relate to them emotionally with real care will the schizoid individual grow and develop the structures needed to manage and enjoy life (Guntrip, 1971).

Returning to the writer Don, I note that despite his being a professional writer, he does not have words for his own inner life. I offer words, such as "dread" and "fear," and he can intellectually acknowledge these are the experiences we are talking about. I watch intently for moments when he is actively feeling rather than talking. Mostly, he feels hopelessness or despair. Understandably, he finds it very difficult to stay in that physiological experience long enough to express it. We touch it—we move on—we return to it—we move on. It is a slow dance between us and between experience and the language of sharing.

CHRISTOPHER BOLLAS

The lineage of the middle school continues to this day with many fine thinkers, analysts, and writers. However, the contemporary who has influenced me the most is Christopher Bollas. Born and first educated in the US, Bollas eventually moved to England, where he became an analyst and a citizen before returning to the US, where he now lives. From the start, Bollas entertained a simultaneous interest in several intellectual arenas, including literature, psychoanalysis, art, social action, and writing, and has written more than a dozen books, most recently on breakdowns and schizophrenia.

One of his most useful ideas is the idea of the "unthought known," which he introduced in 1987. He wrote that the baby's unconscious is created by the actions of the caregiving environment, and these actions are stored, not as thoughts but as ways of being. This is a wonderful description of our unconscious, not a place of repression but a place of lived experience albeit unthought experience. We currently have the work of neuroscience to confirm this understanding of right- and left-brain development, but Bollas eloquently and usefully describes how this works in the subjective psychotherapeutic relationship.

Remember Jack, who falls into bits and pieces when terrorizing images intrude into his awareness? During our time together, Jack's "unthought known" has slowly emerged. Jack had assumed his falling apart was due to his drug abuse history. That is certainly part of the story. But Jack has been "clean" for many years, and yet these frightening images frequently assert themselves into his consciousness. Both of us feel that something other than drug use has been disrupting Jack's going-on-being. And slowly a deeper narrative has emerged. Jack was never safe in his early home life. Both parents were dangerous in different ways: angry, intrusive, and worst of all, unpredictable. Calm could turn to sadism with no notice. Jack finds it difficult to hold this emerging picture of his parents. It is so opposed to their public image as beloved and respected in their church and community. How could these other memories of them be true? He asks me: "Do you believe they are true?"

When Jack trembles with fear or leans toward me with an enraged face, enacting what he experienced as a child, I believe him completely. His body is fully engaged with terror and/or rage. His body has known this experience since the very beginning of his life. Only now can Jack begin to think about these experiences rather than re-live them. Until now, they have been unthought knowns, which found daily expression in his life. As a result, Jack feels chronically unsafe, both when alone and when with others.

Winnicott gave us "transitional objects and transitional space," which are both subjectively and objectively created. Bollas contributes the "transformational object," arguing that the mother changes the baby's state of being with her actions (Bollas, 1987). Her goal is usually to change him from uncomfortable to comfortable, from unhappy to happy. She is his "affect regulator" in the current language of neuroscience. Remember that in the first year of life the baby does not live in the reality of you and me, but rather in the reality of needs and urges. This way of looking at the mother and, by extension, the therapist is very enlightening. Therapists need to be with their patients in such a way that growth or transformation can happen. By the time Bollas is writing, it is assumed that therapy is not an educational, intellectual process; rather, it is an emotional exchange that creates new possibilities, new ways of being. Thinking of the analyst or therapist as a transformational object is very inspiring and also a bit daunting. Bollas writes in a style designed to give the reader the creative experiences he recounts. I find this both attractive and useful.

Bollas further elaborates Winnicott's true self with his own ideas around a "destiny drive," an unconscious force within each of us that is searching for the best environment in which to thrive (Bollas, 1989). For Bollas, the right to pursue our own desires is paramount, for this is where joy and even ecstasy reside. We each have a unique idiom for living life derived from our core self and shaped by our family ways of relating. A meaningful life involves active interaction with the world of people, things, and ideas. Any of these can be transformational objects, enlarging and enriching us.

Bollas, too, is deeply interested in schizoid phenomena and psychosis and has been willing to modify his approach in order to help those in intense need. He is very anti-medication, proclaiming that we all know the wisdom of talking as the most healing medium. He writes in *When the Sun Bursts* of seeing people twice a day for several weeks, or all day many days in a row. His experience is that with this kind of proactive management breakdowns, even psychosis, can be properly worked through, not medicated or avoided (Bollas, 2015).

Bollas challenges each of us to imagine and create our individual lives according to our own desires, not those of someone else. We are essentially alone and must find our personal meaning through this aloneness (Bollas, 1989). Psychoanalysis cannot cure the world of its ills, but it can help each of us create a fresh outlook on our existence, and so make our world vibrate in richer tones and colors. Throughout his extensive writing, he argues that psychoanalysis needs to free itself from the confines of psychology and medicalized psychiatry if it is to fulfill its potential as an agent of meaning and purpose.

Where we are so far: For Freud, psychoanalysis was to be a biological science, and, in that sense, it was to be an objective study of the psyche, the unconscious of his patients. His developmental focus was on what we would now call the triangle of the three-person system, a very mature system in terms of early development in which the child, the mother, and the father all relate each to the other. He believed that the father was the key to civilization by helping the child manage his id impulses, manage his guilt, and come to terms with both his gifts and his limitations.

By the 1940s, the focus in England had shifted dramatically. Instead of the three-person system, many analysts of the time embraced the two-person system, comprising the infant and his caregiver. Instead of focusing on life after ages 5 or 6, they centered on the first years of life. The focus had shifted from the father to the mother as the facilitating environment for development. Rather than an exclusive focus on the inner world, the world of phantasy, and imagination, they recognized the significance of real experiences, and began to wonder what kind of parenting ("environmental provision," in the language of the time) was best for the developing infant. Most importantly, some of them began to realize that the clinical situation presents two subjects, not a subject and an object that is to be studied and cured.

All three strands recounted thus far—Klein's concern with id forces, Anna Freud's insistence on ego functioning and resilience, and the middle group—deepened our understanding of the first years of life and changed the focus of psychoanalysis from drive discharge to relationship and communication. In spite of their tremendous differences, all of these game changers honor Freud as their first and often exclusive intellectual inspiration.

Key concepts Chapter 5

Affect regulator – a current term for talking about how important others are to each of us in maintaining emotional well-being both to soothe and to enliven

Area of creation – Balint's term for the first months of life, wherein the babe is self-contained and full of potential

Basic fault – Balint's term for the early time of life where the world is naturally split into good and bad moments due to the care and failure of care the babe receives. With too much failure of care, the babe does not develop psychically beyond this phase

Benign regression – refers to Balint's belief that the patient needs to regress to a state of trusting dependency on the analyst in order to start over

Capacity for concern – as the babe develops, according to Winnicott, she becomes aware that others exist, and she can care about them and affect them

Central ego – Fairbairn's term for the conscious aspect of the original ego that is stripped of vitality

Collecting impingements – a pattern of relating that assumes others will not treat me well, thereby creating that exact experience

Destiny drive – Bollas' belief that each of us wants to thrive and wants to find the best environment in which to experience our personal essence

Environmental mother – at the beginning of life, the baby experiences the environment as dedicated to meeting his needs, not a person who takes care of him

Exciting object – Fairbairn's term for that aspect of the mother that satisfies and frustrates the baby; sometimes referred to as the frustrating exciting object

Going-on-being – Winnicott's idea that the well cared-for baby experiences few impingements so as to feel herself as alive, continuous, and content

Good enough mother – she is not perfect or rigid, yet holds her baby and his needs in mind most of the time and is willing to fulfill those needs

Harmonious interpenetrating mix-up – Balint's phrase for the ideal relationship between mother and babe; it is effortless and reciprocal

Idealized other – the baby's implicit appraisal of the people he is dependent on, his objects, paired with the central ego

Impingements – anything that disrupts going-on-being

Internal saboteur or sadistic superego – that aspect of the self formed in relation to the rejecting object

Libidinal ego – that aspect of self formed in relation to the exciting object

Lived emotional experience – both Balint and Guntrip emphasized that patients need a real relationship with a real other in order to have a new emotional experience

Love made angry and love made hungry – Guntrip's description of the baby's possibilities when his needs are not met

Malignant regression – Balint's observation that some patients get stuck in dependency and do not move towards mourning and new beginnings

Object mother – the "real" or personal mother who cares for this specific baby

Objective love and hate – the idea that there are aspects of patients that warrant strong approval and strong disapproval, but that offering such direct feedback must be carefully titrated into a useful interpretation

Play – according to Winnicott, in health, play for a child is the simple ability to enjoy and dramatize her inner life; for an adult it is the capacity to use language and other symbols to express the true self without rigidity or anxiety

Pre-moral – at the beginning of life, the baby is not concerned with right and wrong; she is concerned with survival. Concern and morality are developmental achievements within a caring context

Primary love – the first object relationship between the babe and her mother

Primary maternal preoccupation – the state of being of "ordinary" mothers, who are focused primarily on their newborns

Real relationship – in distinction to the transference relationship. Both are ongoing and the "real" relationship is especially important in dealing with pre-Oedipal issues

Rejecting object – Fairbairn's term for that aspect of the mother that frustrates the babe too much of the time

Ruth–ruthless – at the beginning of life, the babe demands that her needs be met immediately—Winnicott referred to this early stage as ruthless and that over time, she develops "ruth"

Schizoid factors – Fairbairn's term for psychic development when needs are not met, and the babe depends too much on his inner fantasies to meet his real needs

Splitting – at the beginning of life when the baby does not live in time it is normal to experience the world as split into good and bad moments; this becomes a pathological stance if there has been too much deprivation, and healthy ambivalence cannot emerge

Spontaneous gestures of emotional creativity – Winnicott's phrase for the natural aliveness within each human being; it is a goal of therapy to restore access to that aliveness

Survival – both mothers with their baby and therapists with their patient need to "survive" negative experiences with neither retaliation nor withdrawal, coming to experience one another as two separate people

Transformational object – Bollas' characterization of the mother as one who transforms the baby's internal and external environment by managing his psychosomatic needs

Transitional objects – soft objects that soothe the baby, reminding him of his mother and her care; they both connect him to her and allow the process of separation

Transitional space – a space that is co-created by mother and babe, by analyst and patient, where change is possible. It is a dimension of living that is neither external nor internal; rather it is both

True self / false self – Winnicott's radical proposal that each individual contained a true self that would never disappear even though it could go into cold storage and be hidden by one or more false selves

Unthought known – Bollas' phrase for the unconscious source of actions and behavior, derived from interacting with others in early life and never thought about

References

Abram, J. (1996) *The Language of Winnicott*. Northvale, NJ: Jason Aronson.
Balint, M. (1957) *The Doctor, His Patient and the Illness*. New York: International Universities.
Balint, M (1965) *Primary Love and Psycho-Analytic Technique*. New York: Liverwright.
Balint, M. (1968, 1979). *The Basic Fault*. New York: Brunner/Mazel.
Bollas, C. (1987) *The Shadow of the Object*. London: Free Association.
Bollas, C. (1989) *Forces of Destiny*. Northvale, NJ: Jason Aronson.
Bollas, C. (2015) *When the Sun Bursts*. New Haven, CT: Yale University.
Davis, M. & Wallbridge, D. (1981) *Boundary and Space*. New York: Brunner/Mazel.
Fairbairn, W.R.D. (1943, 1952) *An Object-Relations Theory of the Personality*. New York: Basic Books.
Gomez, L. (1997) *An Introduction to Object Relations*. London: Free Association Books.
Grosskurth, P. (1986) *Melanie Klein: Her World and Her Work*. New York: Knopf.
Guntrip, H. (1969) *Schizoid phenomena, objects relations and the self*. New York: Basic Books.
Guntrip, H. (1971) *Psychoanalytic Theory, Therapy, and the Self*. New York: Basic Books.
Hazell, J. (1996) *H.J.S. Guntrip: A Psychoanalytical Biography*. London: Free Association Books.
Herman, J. (1992) *Trauma and Recovery*. New York: Basic Books.
Klein, J. (1987) *Our Need for Others and Its Roots in Infancy*. New York: Routledge.
Little, M. (1977) *Psychotic Anxieties and Containment*. Northvale, NJ: Jason Aronson.

Mitchell, S.A. & Black, M. (1995) *Freud and Beyond*. New York: Basic Books.
Phillips, A. (1988) *Winnicott*. Cambridge, MA: Harvard University Press.
Rodman, F.R. (2003) *Winnicott: Life and Work*. Cambridge, MA: Perseus.
Winnicott, D.W. (1947) Hate in the counter-transference. In *Through Paediatrics to Psychoanalysis*. London: Hogarth, 1975.
Winnicott, D.W. (1951) Transitional objects and transitional phenomena. In Winnicott, D.W. (1971) *Playing and Reality*. Harmondsworth, UK: Penguin.
Winnicott, D.W. (1954) Metapsychological and clinical aspects of regression within the psycho-analytical set-up. In *Through Paediatrics to Psychoanalysis*. London: Hogarth, 1975.
Winnicott, D.W. (1956) Primary maternal preoccupation. In *Through Paediatrics to Psychoanalysis*. London: Hogarth, 1975.
Winnicott, D.W. (1960a) Ego distortions in terms of a true and false self. In *Through Paediatrics to Psychoanalysis*. London: Hogarth, 1975.
Winnicott, D.W. (1960b) The theory of the parent–infant relationship. In *The Maturational Processes and the Facilitating Environment*. Madison, CT: International Universities Press, 1965.
Winnicott, D.W. (1963a) From dependence towards independence in the development of the individual. In *The Maturational Processes and the Facilitating Environment*. Madison, CT: International Universities Press, 1965.
Winnicott, D.W. (1963b) The development of the capacity for concern. In *The Maturational Processes and the Facilitating Environment*. Madison, CT: International Universities Press, 1965.
Winnicott, D.W. (1963c) Fear of breakdown. In Winnicott, C., Shepherd, R., & Davis, M. (eds) *Psycho-Analytic Explorations*. London: Karnac, 1989.
Winnicott, D.W. (1964) *The Child, the Family and the Outside World*. Cambridge, MA: Perseus.
Winnicott, D.W. (1967) Mirror role of mother and family in child development. In Winnicott, D.W. (1971) *Playing and Reality*. Harmondsworth, UK: Penguin.
Winnicott, D.W. (1968) The use of an object and relating through identification. In Winnicott, D.W. (1971) *Playing and Reality*. Harmondsworth, UK: Penguin
Winnicott, D.W. (1971) *Playing and Reality*. Harmondsworth, UK: Penguin.
Winnicott, D.W. (1988) *Babies and Their Mothers*. New York: Addison-Wesley.
Young-Bruehl, E. (1988) *Anna Freud: A Biography*. New York: Norton.

6

HEINZ KOHUT

We always need others for our well-being and to create meaning

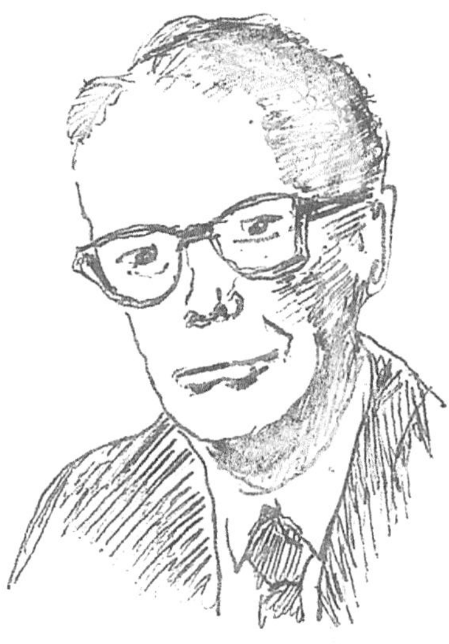

Heinz Kohut

Heinz Kohut (1913–1981) fled Vienna in 1939, interrupting his very assimilated, cultured life, his medical training, and his first analysis. He found his way first to London and then to Chicago, where his rather difficult mother joined him. He finished his medical training and underwent further analysis in order to become a classical psychoanalyst at the Chicago Institute for Psychoanalysis. He was married in 1948 and the couple with their only son established a rhythm of life revolving around, first, his analytic work and then his writing (Strozier, 2001).

Although born in Vienna, and always wanting to stay loyal to Freud, Kohut established a totally different way of looking at analysis and a thoroughly American one. In 1959, he published a paper on empathy, signaling his change away from Freudian drives towards what he would call the self, arguing that it is through empathy that the analyst can truly know the patient (Kohut, 1959). It was a very radical stance. Empathy is quite different from that of an objective knower or observer. The idea of empathy and specifically "empathic immersion" moves the analyst from that neutral objective stance to a much more subjective relationship with his patient. Kohut's technique eventually included what he called empathic immersion and "vicarious introspection." Both address the question: What is the world like from another's point of view? This change in perspective allowed him to imagine the other's meanings and significance rather than attempt to fit the other into a particular belief or theory (Kohut, 1984).

Empathy

Neurobiologically, empathy is a survival tool that allows us to inhabit the feelings of others. We now know that mirror neurons exist in the brain that allow us to mimic others' movements and predict their actions. Our brain is designed to read faces at birth. Empathy expands both our awareness and our capacity to connect. It also is a skill that can be practiced. Therapeutically, empathy does not mean "being nice." Rather, it means responding to the other's emotional needs as understood in this moment (Siegel, 2007).

However, it is with the publication of his first book in 1971, *The Analysis of the Self*, that the extent of the radical shift in Kohut's thinking became totally apparent to the analytic community of the time. No longer focused on the inner Freudian biological battles of drives and the guilt over forbidden wishes, he became absorbed with developmental deficits, personal isolation and alienation, and the struggle to create meaning. Kohut completely changed our understanding of narcissism and wrote that these more fragile and less mature clients could be helped. In his *Analysis of the Self*, the developing child needs to be the center of realistic parental love and limits. He believes in a much stronger need than that of the average expectable environment of the middle school. For Freud, the infant was absorbed in primary narcissism and omnipotent thought, and he maintained that in adults this immature grandiosity must be confronted. In his clinical work, Kohut found that confronting narcissistic individuals with their shortcomings was not helpful; they fell into deep inadequacy and painful humiliation, even despair. They plummeted from omnipotent superiority to dangerous fragility. Unrealistic narcissism provided spark and excitement but no ability to love and connect. Kohut believed that narcissistic individuals created an "as if" self because their authentic human self was never seen and validated. Their parents had organized the child into serving their needs rather than they themselves joyfully meeting the needs of their undeveloped child (Kohut, 1971).

The impact of the *Analysis of the Self* on the New York psychoanalytic community was slow but, gradually, most rejected its foundational premise that developmental trauma is the defining event and that the child needs a long period immersed in idealization, pushing drive theory and the Oedipal triangle into a secondary role. Once seen as a possible heir to the throne of American psychoanalysis, Kohut was now in conflict with all of these figures, including Anna Freud (Strozier, 2001). The psychoanalytic community has always been tough on innovators. It has been quick to extrude people and ideas that do not meet the litmus test of "Would Freud have agreed with this?" And certainly, Kohut's thinking could no longer be seen as in agreement with Freud.

However, it is in his second book, *The Restoration of the Self*, that Kohut totally breaks with tradition while staying in intense conversation with Freud. Kohut had already developed his own language to describe his theories. One is "self-object," which first of all refers to a child's parents and then to others who support the solidity, continuity, and positive value of the developing self (Kohut, 1971). The self-object is a person, or an aspect of a person, used as a function to create inner stability, continuity, and well-being. Over time, Kohut maintained that we need self-objects and the meaning they create throughout our lives, and to emphasize their important meaning in his theory, he changed the spelling to "selfobject." For him, we are never going to achieve clear autonomy and separation. Rather, the goal is deeper and deeper engagement and connection with our important others. Intimacy is the source of happiness, not hyper-independence.

Kohut completely revamped our understanding of narcissism, conceiving of these struggles as part of developmental arrest rather than a defense. The tragedy of the narcissist is his own lack of wholeness, his lack of feeling real. Although he tries to hide his despair, he knows in his heart that he is "less than," somehow inferior or fragmented. His self-experience is that, "fundamentally, I am flawed." For Kohut, this is the result of self-object failure, the parental environment itself is the problem. He called this focus "tragic man," in distinction to Freud's "guilty man" (Kohut, 1977).

Freud gave us the aphorism that the key to a good life is the ability to love and to work. True, no doubt, but for Kohut the good life also must include the ability to feel joy and inner vitality as well as pride in our own creations. He encouraged therapists to focus on each individual's strengths and gifts, not only his or her defenses and limits (Kohut, 1984). He proclaimed that he was less interested in interpretation and more interested in reconstruction (Kohut, 1977).

Empathy was the seminal theme for Kohut from his 1959 article to his last lecture a week before he died. He called his method the introspective-empathic method (Strozier, 2001). At first, Kohut defined "empathy" as vicarious introspection. Over time, his view of empathy became ever more complex and intersubjective. He acknowledged its biological roots were required for survival. But it is much more than that. Ongoing empathy reveals that the other cares and that the individual is worth caring for. Over time, it proves that ruptures can be repaired. It is required for emotional and intellectual development. It is the foundation for faith and trust—first in people and then in life. By the end of his life, he believed that empathy cures.

Kohut held "empathic immersion" as an ideal and fully realized that we don't/can't live up to that ideal. He argued for the importance of being empathetic to the feelings and needs of the other, especially when we, as therapists, fail or disappoint our clients. We need to empathize with their disappointment at our failures, acknowledge it, and hopefully repair the situation (Kohut, 1984). He was carefully critical of his more classical colleagues, saying their technique put them in a bind: to be warm and human would be to break the rules and engender guilt (Strozier, 2001).

Kohut also rewrote the book on "narcissistic rage"—certainly one of his most valuable contributions to analytic thinking and clinical work. Freud saw this rage as part of the death instinct. Kohut felt that free and wholesome aggression was necessary and could serve healthy ambitions. By his reasoning, if there is inappropriate rage, it must protect an inability to appropriately assert oneself or to express one's needs. From this perspective, when we therapists investigate rage—even in its milder forms—we usually find we are talking about a blending of past and present. Rage emanates from the used or abandoned child within the angry adult, from the child who was impotent, who could not get his needs met in that historical environment and became convinced that he could never get those needs met (Kohut, 1972).

At the beginning of life, we are all narcissistically inclined, intent on getting what we need first to survive and then to thrive. In our childhood fantasies, we live in a world of superheroes and super forces without human perspective. We believe we are capable of anything and deserve everything. Sometimes we have good enough parents who protect us and teach us to manage these fantasies; sometimes we have parents who fail us occasionally; and sometimes we have parents who fail us consistently. Over time, Kohut hypothesized that children need three different kinds of parental experiences in order to mature. They need a "mirror" to reflect their inner emotional states, thus supporting their expansive narcissistic states and solidifying their innate sense of vitality and aliveness. They need someone to "idealize," permitting merger with powerful others, thereby creating safety, inner calmness, and infallibility. And they need someone with whom to "twin," saying in essence, "I am like you and we are both good." For Kohut and analysts in his lineage, it is important to enhance these states at the beginning of life and simply let reality slowly do its transformative work. In such an unfolding, the child builds inner resilience and an internal secure home base (Kohut,1977).

So, in Kohut's understanding, gathering a whole sense of self starts with the parent mirroring the child's healthy grandiosity. This, in turn, generates healthy pride and healthy assertiveness. When the parents do not or cannot perform that necessary function, Kohut wrote that the consequences are shame and rage, both of which disorganize the personality or sense of self (Kohut, 1972). Thus, he started the conversation within the analytic community around shame as differentiated from guilt. (Several others had made that distinction on the importance of shame before him, but this critical topic was not integrated into mainstream thinking for several decades.) Several self psychologists have expanded the importance of shame as a felt sense of diminishment and deficit, a sense of falling from grace and wholeness. Clinically, understanding that exaggerated, inappropriate narcissism hides a profound sense of shame is critical to healing this form of suffering (Morrison, 1984).

Kohut translated these developmental needs into varieties of transferences with his patients, especially his narcissistic patients. His technique became that of working with the three self-object transferences. Given a responsive, often non-interpretive environment, he believed that each individual would naturally move towards their own unique, meaningful goals. For him, the analytic relationship needs to be supportive in very specific ways. In the so-called "mirroring transference," the analyst continually reflects to the patient that his emotional states are seen, registered, and valued. This allows the patient to feel "real" in the same way Winnicott's holding environment allowed his patients to feel real. The "idealizing transference" encourages the patient to reconnect with his agency, his innate ability to act on his own behalf. And the "alter ego" or "twinship transference" reassures the patient that "we are essentially alike and that we share a sensibility about what it means to be a living human being" (Kohut, 1971, 1977).

His model acknowledges that the patient requires extended immersion in these transference states in order for arrested, authentic vitality to re-ignite. Rather than offering interpretations from a separate point of view, the analyst allows himself to be used as a function that can be internalized and slowly transmute the patient's arrested development. It is important to always assume and respect the patient's desire to grow and mature. For self psychologists, the Freudian aggressive and sexual pressures remain secondary.

In spite of initially wishing to only extend Freud, Kohut fundamentally re-conceptualized the analytic project from a management of id drives through ego functions to one of restarting innate development, organically opening the doors to internal coherence, vitality, and creativity (1977). In *Restoration of the Self*, Kohut wrote that there are many selves within each of us, highlighting that the Freudian ego was never going to be in charge and at peace. Somewhat confusingly, he decided that we need to think simultaneously of the idea of the self as the center of the psychological universe and, at the same time, the self is a content of mental apparatus as in Freud's structural model. For Kohut, the "I" is the self, and the self makes no sense without its selfobjects. There can be no self without a context. Self ↔ selfobject. Self ↔ context.

In Kohut's mature writings, his notion of tragic man is most vivid. All of us must mourn unrealized dreams, whether created by personal family life or the impersonal forces of history. Despair is the logical response to un-mirrored ambitions and missing ideals. The self must struggle to keep continuity, to resist fragmentation in our modern world. These are very existential themes, clearly different from the Freudian project.

Kohut favored complexity, humanism, and contextualism, maintaining that our own point of view is a perspective that is fundamentally shaped and limited by our personal history and emotional conviction (Kohut, 1984). From the viewpoint of self psychology, we need good parents, we need connection throughout our lives, and we need to create meaning and authenticity. The first two are prerequisites for the third.

In spite of the Holocaust and his personal relationship to it, Kohut was essentially an optimist and believed in the goodness of people and of Life. For him, even tragic circumstances can birth creativity (Strozier, 2001).

I cannot leave this discussion of Kohut without comparing him with Kernberg, as both wrote so extensively on narcissism. Their differences may be due in part to their definitions of narcissism, especially regarding the role of aggression in narcissistic disorders. I have already mentioned Kernberg in terms of his more Kleinian orientation. He roots pathological narcissism as much in constitution as in a developmental context and suggests that it is on a continuum with borderline disorders. For Kernberg, the narcissist has excessive aggression, which must be confronted in order to be integrated. Furthermore, his patient population often requires group work and/or hospitalization in order to be helped.

For Kohut, the failures of the environment are the main source of the narcissistic dilemma. For him, the issue is developmental arrest and, in order to heal, the individual needs to express these archaic needs within the new and safe framework provided by the analyst (Kohut, 1971). Unlike Kernberg, these issues are not instinctual wishes that must be renounced. They are missed developmental needs, which must be revisited and understood. Stephen Mitchell, who will be introduced in the next chapter, provides some resolution to this clash of theory and technique Mitchell, 1993; Mitchell & Black, 1995).

Kohut influences how I sit with and interact with virtually all of those who come to me. His emphasis on empathy and his notion of empathic immersion are the foundation of our work together. Mary's envy, Jess' need for quiet and time, Jack's terror, and Don's isolation all respond to the foundation of emotionally "being with" that Kohut advocates. They each need vitalization some of the time and calming at other times, but those are possible only in the context of the connection provided by the attuned mirroring.

Kohut's theories remained imbedded in the traditional one-person psychology. The analyst is the "parent" to the patient's "child." This is very much in the tradition of the doctor as authority and the patient as the problem. Kohut never abandoned that position; however, his empathic immersion—with its insistence that the analyst seek to experience the world of another—sets the stage for a subject-to-subject field of inquiry.

GEORGE ATWOOD AND ROBERT STOLOROW: INTERSUBJECTIVITY

Kohut's self psychology has its own branches, including the very important work known as "intersubjectivity." I cite George Atwood and Robert Stolorow as two of the current seminal contributors to this way of thinking. Their intersubjective model incorporates both Kohut and systems theory. Systems theory was first introduced into psychology by the family therapists. With the introduction of systemic thinking to Kohut's empathic immersion, the focus of the analysis becomes the fully contextual interaction of two subjectivities acknowledging the "reciprocal mutual influence" between patient and analyst (Stolorow & Atwood, 1992). Realizing and accepting that not only is the analyst influencing the patient but also the patient is constantly influencing the analyst reorients the focus of analysis. Reciprocal mutual influence represents a much fuller and more complex idea than that of transference–countertransference. Countertransference has typically been seen as a problem to be solved. Reciprocal mutual influence is to be acknowledged as universal and used as part of the treatment.

Intersubjectivity as a field of psychoanalysis has come to mean the relational contexts in which all experience occurs, at whatever developmental level: linguistic or pre-linguistic, shared or solitary. An "intersubjective field" is defined as any system formed by interacting experiential worlds. For Stolorow and Atwood, the intersubjective field is more than a mode of experiencing and a sharing of experience. It challenges the belief of the isolated brain-mind within the skin of one person. Furthermore, it is the contextual precondition for having any experience at all. Within these dynamic intersubjective systems, the outcomes of developmental or therapeutic processes are emergent and unknown, not programmed or prescribed. More doors are open; more is possible; and, at the same time, more is unknown and unknowable.

Systems theory

Systems theory developed separately from psychoanalysis. The idea of a system was imported from other branches of science and only much later applied to psychotherapy. Systemic therapists are interested in working with the entire family, seeing the family as the essential defining context of human beings. An important change within this model is the shift from linear cause-and-effect thinking to circular thinking, where communication—both verbal and nonverbal—operates in feedback loops. The notion of the feedback loop is a better metaphor for human experience than mechanistic linear thinking, and it has influenced all forms of psychotherapy (Ruesch & Bateson, 1951).

Dan and Jess represent two examples of my personal experience with reciprocal mutual influence. Both of them are quiet and withdrawn as they enter my office, but they affect me very differently. When Jess enters, I find myself leaning back in my chair breathing calmly and my mind relaxed into attentive waiting for her to find her words. With Dan, I am slightly anxious, learning forward, attentive in a different way. Dan wants words from me, and I do not know what words will come to me. I must wait and trust that Dan and I will find the words that will connect us. In both situations, nonverbal feedback between us is continuous. I want to pay attention to my client's body and words as well as my inner states in order to stay both present and connected.

In response to the loss of his beloved wife, Stolorow (2007) has written extensively and personally on recovering and not recovering from trauma and loss. He asks us to hold both as ongoing without anything that might be called closure. This is a very different take on mourning and closer to my experience both with my clients and with myself. Inner boundaries are both necessary and not neat and fixed. Stolorow's personal disclosures represent a seismic shift in the psychoanalytic literature and, for me, a welcome one. Historically, psychoanalysis has focused on becoming a science and staying objective. Before Stolorow, with few exceptions, the closest thing to personal disclosure was the discussion of countertransference and the very human need for love by some in the British middle school.

As co-authors, Stolorow and Atwood have written most helpfully on the intersubjective process, both child–parent and patient–analyst and developmental arrest (1992; Stolorow & Lachman, 1980). Following Kohut, "developmental arrest" refers to the consequences of not meeting the three early transactional childhood needs: to be mirrored, to be allowed to idealize, and to twin with the powerful parents. The deprived adult lives in a less than optimal way, looking for her archaic needs to be met in current situations. For the intersubjectivists, analytic work is embedded in the process between the two individuals. Framed within systems thinking, what will happen between those two individuals is both unique and unknown. It is emergent—the specific co-creation of these two individuals. In this model, to work contextually means to work both in the present, between patient and analyst, and at the same time developmentally, with the patient's past. It is a delicate balance to stay in the present while maintaining an ongoing sensibility to both participants' past, present, and future. We all have come from somewhere and each of us is on our way to somewhere.

Just acknowledging these ideas—emergent and unknown, not programmed and prescribed—puts both analyst and patient into a quite different way of being together. Yes, they are two separate and different people with different intentions and needs — one suffering, one hoping to alleviate that suffering—however, the analyst's subjective sense of both himself and his task has been re-written completely. Now, we have the task—or might we even say the faith—that by being together, fully present, something of value will emerge. This is not a question of uncovering id impulses, the envy, or the greed, nor is it a question of avoiding such painful negative feelings. For this analyst, it is a question of sitting together, staying curious, asking informed questions, and waiting with hope, welcoming whatever needs to emerge.

BERNARD BRANDCHAFT

Bernard Brandchaft, (1916–2013) is another American contributor to the intersubjective school. After medical school, his intellectual journey started with ego psychology (as was the case with most Americans). Next, he studied with British object-relations theorists Winnicott and Bion; then Kohut; and later, wrote with Atwood and Stolorow, embracing the intersubjective model. His last contribution was facilitated by two of his colleagues and is his strongest statement of a fully intersubjective form of therapy.

Towards an Emancipatory Psychoanalysis (2010) placed psychoanalysis firmly into the two-subject world. All of his basic assumptions are two-person. For example: All intrapsychic phenomena are co-determined. Whatever is going on stems from the interactions of two people. And further, careful attempts to understand what both have contributed to any misunderstanding will advance the therapeutic process. Finally, both people are attempting to both protect and develop self-experience.

Like Stolorow and Atwood, he believed that each patient and analyst form a unique, inextricable psychological system. A key to connection is to search for what is genuine in the words of one another, trusting that the patient will find ways of expressing his suffering. Through such dialogue, each will discover or create meaning. For him learning is always a joint process.

Brandchaft wrote clearly that the analyst may be as changed by the encounter with this specific other as the patient is. Winnicott noted this as well by noting that his patients paid him to learn, even though he remained within the traditional stance of doctor to patient. Brandchaft was more radical, encouraging humility and fallibility on the part of the analyst.

Pathological accommodation

"Pathological accommodation" is the internalized requirement that an individual must distort his own needs to protect the crucial attachment bond. Brandchaft points out that this applies equally to the analyst, in both his personal and professional lineage. Pathological accommodation can be summarized by the following: If I choose for myself or if I do not submit to your humiliating demand, you will abandon me, shun me, or despise me; then, I will finally and forever be alone (Brandchaft et al., 2010). Any family system experiences these choices daily, hopefully in a non-pathological form. When does one member accommodate another in order to spend time together, or keep the peace, and when is it important that each do what they are being called to do? Accommodation becomes a problem when it is internalized as a part of "me"—I must accommodate you, I cannot choose for myself. Once pathological accommodation becomes a part of internal organization, we can only live reactively, never creatively. In Brandchaft's view, each of our subjective worlds originated in interaction with the external world. Therefore, it will be the real therapeutic relationship, not insights or interpretations, that transforms this distortion into a more wholesome balance, where each individual can get some of their needs met without the attachment bond being threatened (Brandchaft et al., 2010).

Brandchaft suggests that when we meet these structures of pathological accommodation in our patients, we can infer a particular parental stance: If you are not what I need you to be, you don't exist for me. He called this "relational trauma." The suffering is acute, paradoxical, and unsolvable because the caregiver and traumatizing one are one and the same. Within this way of being, Brandchaft found the following layers: compulsive craving for love and affirmation, self-hatred, feelings of worthlessness, and despair at the utter failure to bring joy into another's life. As a result, both life and the self become meaningless, worthless, and empty. His is clearly a two-person system; he does not think about the struggles of his patient without wondering about the real dynamics between that patient and his significant others, that patient and himself.

Brandchaft wrote that rebellion can protect the fragile shards of true self-experience. Within the therapeutic hour, it is important for therapists to pay attention to things that irritate us, such as lateness, not paying on time, and the need for constant rescheduling. Through careful, nonjudgmental inquiry via Kohut's empathic immersion, we can find the meaning in these "resistances," and find the organizing principles, the pathological accommodations stored in the pre-reflexive unconscious. Each irritating action is a code covering pathological accommodation with reflexive hyper-independence. His approach provides still another way of understanding and working with the enactment of narcissistic rage and the need for revenge to balance the past in the present.

Brandchaft's ideal was to create what he called "emancipatory therapy." He wrote admiringly of Winnicott's journey to free himself from Klein and the biologically innate drive system she espoused. He was very familiar with Winnicott's concepts of the true/false self and how compliance stifles the "real." Yet he took these concepts much further. He was keenly aware that some re-traumatization within the therapeutic dyad was inevitable. Balancing the need to not re-traumatize with the need to create both space and connection for each individual demonstrates his grasp of the continual need to accommodate the other in order to preserve life-giving connection.

Resistance

For Freud, resistance was an attempt to evade and cover up impulses from the analyst. Kohut saw it as an attempt to protect a fragile self from fragmentation. Brandchaft insists that we must trust that the patient is guiding us to engage in the struggle against self-destroying compliance. In this concept alone, we can see the evolution of analysis. We may not agree, but it is there for the conversation.

With any psychotherapy that is based on creating a safe, vitalizing relationship, the possibility of both re-traumatization and pathological accommodation are continuous, as these are the two sides of impingement. Any time two separate people are in connection it is possible that we hurt each other or overly comply with each other. As I noted above, we must accommodate somewhat in order to stay connected, and what is too much?

Holding the intersubjective stance as a key force for helping and healing means that I, the therapist, must not only be aware of my inner thoughts and feelings but also must be aware of when I have enacted something with a patient and be able to repair that disruption.

Jess continuously over-accommodates, both the people in her life and me. The impact on me is that I must move slowly with her. For example, do I ask her to change her session time? Will her answer come only from that distorted accommodating place within her or from a genuine place of ease? Furthermore, when I say something too sharp or even perhaps shaming, she will never mention it to me. When I reflect on our time together I sometimes realize that what I said could be experienced that way and I need to find another way. I must find a way to re-enter that moment between us and explore it at a later time.

Kohut's self psychology and the evolution of psychoanalysis into an intersubjective model has radically changed the playing field of American psychoanalysis. Drives, inner conflicts, and repression are still part of the psychic structure, but the formative issues are now interpersonal, parental failure, psychic deficit, and relational trauma. When the environment could not meet the needs of the baby with pleasure and delight, the budding sense of self suffered and became distorted in innumerable ways. Furthermore, this school of thought has influenced many contemporary researchers. I will catalogue a few of the most visible who have had the greatest influence on the field.

DANIEL STERN

American Daniel Stern, (1934–2012) contributed to the analytic project both as a researcher and as a clinician. His research contributions have been invaluable to me and the therapeutic community. Kohut's theories gained immeasurable credibility when Stern published his 1985 book, *The Interpersonal World of the Infant*. Through many rigorous studies in his laboratory, Stern confirmed that, from the very beginning of life, the infant oscillates between intense connection and budding differentiation. He used the infant's ability to communicate through sucking and head turning to ask questions the tiny baby could answer. His phases of development are different from those of Mahler, and they are rooted in what he calls the "emergent senses of self," which are present as biological givens or potentials from the very beginning of life. These are: agency, affectivity, cohesion, and history. Every human being develops and inhibits these inbuilt potentials. His research, like that of Bowlby, has influenced all of psychotherapy and psychoanalysis but it was most fully and quickly embraced by the self psychology community.

Stern suggests that a "core" or physical sense of self also is available at birth, wherein the infant recognizes separate bodies but cannot yet grasp the psychological significance of his physical experiences. (For me this is analogous to Ogden's autistic-contiguous position.) At around nine months, a "subjective sense of self" emerges, and the infant recognizes the differing minds of self and others. Following this, the two modes of experience co-exist: a pre-subjective core, or physical sense of self, alongside a subjective or psychological self.

As soon as the infant discovers that both he and his mother have unique separate psychological lives, he experiences a need for bridges of empathic connection. Mahler first documented this in what she called her "rapprochement phase," but Stern looked at it somewhat differently. The infant realizes that, while two minds can enjoy sharing, they also can differ, and this first awareness of psychic difference leads to new anxieties about conflict, separation, and abandonment. If the caregiver responds with increased attunement at this critical juncture, the infant goes on to be curious about the newly recognized, distinctive mind of the other. But without heightened attunement at this point, the infant's natural curiosity can be swamped by anxiety. For Stern, the terrible twos are not a developmental given and, if the parents can stay attuned both to the toddler and to themselves, development can proceed without great ruptures and drama.

For the self psychologists, this recognition of relational capacities at birth translated into a greater emphasis on the affective components of the psychoanalytic cure. For them, affect is the connecting link among all the qualities of engagement, replacing drives as the primary human motivator. The sense of self is organized around affective interpersonal experience. But this organization can emerge and remain open and flexible only when affective experience is adequately regulated through the self–self-object relationship.

As a therapist, Stern (2004) privileges feelings over thoughts and the current exchange between therapist and client over understanding history. His detailed understanding of the therapeutic process weaving past and present explicates both his formidable body of research on mother–baby dyads and his sensitive clinical style.

BEATRICE BEEBE AND FRANK LACHMANN

In New York, Beatrice Beebe, and Frank Lachmann, publish on their own, together, and with others. What has been most valuable to me is their research on the mother–infant couple and its application to psychotherapy with adults (Beebe & Lachmann, 2002). In her basic research, Beebe uses video cameras trained simultaneously on the faces of the mother and the child. Then she splices the two together, presenting a split-frame image with a micro timer running underneath. Through the use of this technology, she documents the interactions between the pair that are invisible to the naked eye. For example, by watching a video of the infant, we see him frown and his head droop, but we do not see what might have caused that reaction. To our naked eye, the mother sounds OK and her face seems OK. It would be easy to assume that the cause of the frown and the head droop was strictly internal. When Beebe slows and splices the tape showing both mother and baby at the same time, we can see the fleeting moment of disgust on the mother's face that precedes the infant's withdrawal. On the basis of millions of such interactions, Beebe asserts confidently that both partners of the dyad are always unconsciously working on the process of fitting together. Among others, her research has demonstrated how both consciously and non-consciously attuned we are to the human face. Whether this leads to "pathological accommodation" or enlivened vitality is a co-creation of the mother–baby fit. Most would agree that the mother, the adult mind, is the more responsible for the overall emotional tone of the relationship; however, we should not discount how difficult some babies are. The concept of the fit is really key.

One of the key concepts for psychological healing elucidated by Beebe and Lachmann is the importance of the "cycle of rupture and repair" (Beebe & Lachmann, 2002). Like the therapist and patient, baby and mother can misunderstand each other or be angry at each other or wish to separate and withdraw in various ways. In spite of our best efforts as therapists we can misattune to the other and it is important to remember that this is both inevitable and even necessary. If these misattunements are repaired and understood, the result will be increased awareness, actually strengthening the bond between us. Beebe and Lachman can point out on the videotape where the mother learns the signal of her baby after one of these misses or where the baby figures out something about the reactions of her mother. Fusion and perfection are not possible but learning from our mistakes certainly is.

Available videos

In today's world many researchers and even therapists are posting videos of their work allowing them to reach a much broader audience. Beebe and her students have posted such work allowing us to see what she sees in her micro-tracking experiments. Another fabulous three-minute video has been posted by Edward Tronick, a Boston baby researcher, called the still-face experiment (2007). This video elucidates how in less than a minute, the infant collapses physically and psychologically when, at the request of the experimenter, the mother quits interacting with her baby and instead lets her face go still.

When Jack is not falling apart in terror, he can be very impatient with me when I don't "get" what he means right away. I experience him as speaking in fragments, making allusions to random events as if we have talked about them many times before. He often ends his speech with, "You know, right?" When I reply to say I don't know, Jack is either crestfallen or dismissive. When he is dismissive, I experience the defensive contempt—I should know without being told just like someone should have known his needs when he was very young. Jack was raised by nannies hired by his deeply self-involved parents. They did not have time for him and they let him know it. As an adult, they are only interested in his accomplishments, preferably in some public arena, such as politics. Jack is still struggling with the developmental wounds Kohut writes of so eloquently. He needs the function of a strong, clear mirror in order to find himself. My "not getting" him, means to him that he is not connected to me—another abandonment, another loss. We will repeat this cycle many times: my interrupting by not knowing, his frustration, our mutual attempts to re-connect. Beebe and Lachmann's rupture and repair cycle is building a bond of trust between us. He knows that I will not always get him, but he is beginning to experience that I care enough and am curious enough to figure out what is needed in the immediate situation and what kind of attention or acknowledgment would create safety and be enlivening.

Projective identification / intersubjective thinking

We have now arrived at a very different understanding of the process that one-person theorists call "projective identification." Projective identification is linear: The patient's hidden and unconscious intent causes the analyst's visceral state. But in intersubjective thinking, we are all imbedded in complex systems. Each of us is contributing to the interaction all the time. We both have unknown and unconscious intents. Once we enter into systems thinking and the idea of the intersubjective field, we have to relinquish or at least modify linear cause and effect. We affect each other continuously, both verbally and nonverbally, consciously and non-consciously, creating a trajectory that is not predictable from any one element seen in isolation. This is now assumed to be a completely normal ongoing process among all connected human beings.

With all of these changes in assumptions, the analyst is now required to look at his own contributions to the system. He can no longer assume neutrality and that he can contain his countertransference. As on Beebe's split screens, both parties are affecting each other microsecond by microsecond. We know from Paul Ekman's research (2003) that we are prewired to respond unconsciously to the expressions on the face of others and do so both knowingly and unknowingly all the time. We don't need to assume unconscious intentionality or projective mechanisms. We do need to assume an interactive flow between patient and analyst, with the analyst monitoring his own contributions as well as the contributions co-created between the dyad.

DONNA ORANGE

Before leaving Kohut's lineage, I want to mention the contemporary Donna Orange, of both New York and Rome, as a representative of the group of psychoanalysts who are turning to philosophy for further inspiration in their effort to relieve psychological suffering. In contrast, American psychiatry of today is primarily interested in biological solutions to psychological suffering. Through that lens, human suffering has been thoroughly "medicalized" and many assume that a pill can cure a patient's problems in living his life. Some forms of suffering like intense depressions and anxieties can only be relieved by neuro-chemical intervention, and it must be said that, for many, medications are a true godsend. On the other hand, feeling real and valuable and finding meaning and goals can only be created, or perhaps more accurately co-created, in a human context.

Orange writes passionately that studying philosophy will help us clinically. Specifically, I have been inspired by her writings on hermeneutics and about specific philosophers and how they can influence our clinical style.

Hermeneutics

Stemming from the Greek messenger of the gods Hermes, hermeneutics is the study of interpretation. Hermes carried messages from the divine to the human, and hermeneutics was first a study of sacred texts. Over time it became a general dialogical understanding of both philosophy and the social sciences. Orange proposes that it should become a part of what she calls an ethical clinical sensibility for clinicians, of all persuasions. How do we approach the patient, what are our basic assumptions? (Orange, 2011)

In her study of philosophy, Orange (2011) offers the "hermeneutics of trust" and the "hermeneutics of suspicion" as stances of the therapist. To approach the other with trust is to assume common ground: We work, and play, and search for meaning. The hermeneutics of trust assumes goodwill and trustworthiness, not that everything is clear and obvious. This is in distinction to the hermeneutics of suspicion, which is advocated by Freud and others, especially Klein and Kernberg. Here, concealment is assumed, and the clinician must get under the surface meaning to the truth. Freud's interest in negation—when the patient means the opposite of what he is saying—is among the clearest examples of this clinical stance. When Mitchell (in the next chapter) challenges Winnicott and Kohut suggesting they receive the other in an unquestioning way, thereby perpetuating the old ways of being, he is claiming his place in the hermeneutics of suspicion.

Two of Orange's (2010) philosophers, Martin Buber (1878–1965) and Emmanuel Levinas (1906–1995), also have deeply informed my clinical work. Martin Buber has been a guide for many years. More recently, Emmanuel Levinas has provided inspiration.

Both Buber and Levinas were European Jews who survived the Nazi attempt to take over Europe and eradicate all Jews. Given that background, their formulations are even more remarkable. Buber (1958) is rightly famous for his statement that, within human relationships, we must treat others as a "thou," not an object to be used in any way. He wrote that love is the responsibility of an "I" for a "thou." He spoke of symmetry and connection between equals. He warned that while we may believe we are communicating in a real and attuned manner, we often are still leaving the other out of the dialogue and continuing in our personal self-absorption. Only when we can filter these distractions entirely will we create the "I–thou," allowing direct and meaningful communication. Buber knew well that these encounters are rare, even perhaps more of an ideal than an ongoing human possibility.

According to Orange, Levinas took this position a radical step further. His ethics were formed by four years in a Nazi work camp, a situation of utter humiliation and de-humanization. Yet, he still proposed that the only ethical position in life is a radically asymmetrical relationship of infinite responsibility to the other. He came to the conclusion that we must always treat the other as a "face," not as something to be studied. This irreducible face always transcends our concepts, representations, and ideas. The other presents me with an infinite demand for protection and care. The face says, "you shall not kill me," and "you shall not allow me to die alone."

Orange points out that, for Buber, the "between" is primary. For Levinas, the face of the suffering other is primary. Furthermore, she believes that when we are present to another, we are emotionally available, which is part of the ethical attitude of proximity and readiness to respond to the other that makes for good psychotherapy of any kind.

We are now firmly in the realm of what can be called modern psychoanalysis. Today theory proposes that the therapeutic encounter is that of two subjects interacting, not knowing exactly what will unfold at any given moment. This in no way denies all the previous layers of the psyche that have been discovered and described over the last 150 years. Depending on training and orientation, each clinician will look for drives or guilt, or schizoid factors, pathological narcissism, lack of vitalization, or any of the other theoretical stances outlined here. In practice, modern psychoanalysis is more often face-to-face, recognizing how important that social, nonverbal connection is. Today, the clinician will more often be asking questions, offering fewer interpretations. There is a much greater emphasis on "being with" rather than interpretations and insights as the healing force. The frame is still crucial. Self-disclosure is frowned upon although the analyst presents him- or herself as a real human being who can make mistakes rather than only as a wise authority.

Our next two chapters, on relational psychoanalysis and attachment theory, will further ground us in this modern stance. As we will see, relational theory insists that there are two living separate people in the room and that the most fruitful conversation focuses on the present exchange between the two participants, while the attachment lineage proposes that growth can happen only when the container is safe enough. In both stances the quality of the relationship is the key to healing and health.

Key concepts Chapter 6

Co-determined – a modern assumption that relationships including analytic relationships involve emotional, nonverbal, and verbal input from all parties

Core sense of self – Stern's phrase for the baby's development when his emergent senses of self are mirrored and allowed to flourish

Cycle of rupture and repair – Beebe and Lachmann's description of the pattern between mother and baby of attuning, misattuning, distress, and repair of that distress

Developmental arrest – within self psychology, pathology is created when the basic needs of a developing infant are not met, and growth is curtailed

Emancipatory therapy – Brandchaft's theory and practice of analysis that emphasizes pathological accommodation and existential freedom

Emergent senses of self – Stern's research-based observations that each infant contains the capacity for agency, affectivity, cohesion, and self-history

Empathic immersion – Kohut's analytic technique encouraging the analyst to see the world through the needs and feelings of his patient; a subjective stance

Empathy – our inbuilt capacity to emotionally understand others and therefore to connect with them. An important curative term in the lexicon of self psychology

Face – for Levinas, the face holds an ethical call to offer the "other" infinite compassion and care

Hermeneutics – a term in philosophy and later psychoanalysis describing the science of interpretation, noting that the lens we use for interpreting others determines what follows

Hermeneutics of suspicion – Orange's term for the classical Freudian lens; things are not as they appear to be

Hermeneutics of trust – Orange's term for the lens humanistic psychology and some others employ when sitting with patients; the patient will unfold in her own time when provided with safety and care

I–thou – Buber's injunction that we treat each "other" as a sacred, important being; he also realized it was an ideal

Idealize – to hold in high regard; specifically for Kohut, the need children have to see their parents as good so that they can internalize those strengths and capabilities

Idealizing transference – Kohut's belief that it is important for many patients to idealize their analyst in order to incorporate new positive aspects

Intersubjectivity – the complex field of interaction between analyst and patient creating emotional connection as opposed to a subject and object of study

Mirror – a first basic need of the baby that his inner life, his feelings be mirrored by the face, tone, and sounds of the mother

Mirroring transference – a basic need of a patient to have his emotions reflected back to him by the analyst thus validating the reality and necessity of those emotions

Narcissism – a term used to describe a continuum of characteristics from healthy agency to pathological self-centeredness

Narcissistic rage – rage that stems from feeling intense humiliation; it includes the need to destroy the cause of that humiliation

Pathological accommodation – Brandchaft's theory that unconscious compliant attachment is a major source of both pathology and suffering

Psychology of the self – Kohut's theories as distinct from Freud's drive theory

Reciprocal mutual influence – Hartmann's idea that the baby and the mother are affecting each other and need each other continually; important to both self psychology and relational psychology

Relational trauma – also referred to as "strain" trauma; when the parent does not attune and mirror the child, the child develops a set of defenses to survive, foreclosing the possibility of spontaneous, joyful living

Self-object – Kohut's term for any person who is used to help create a sense of self; self-objects are needed throughout life in order to thrive

Shame – a felt sense of diminishment and deficit, a sense of falling from grace and wholeness; increasingly a focus of clinical work

Subjective sense of self – as development proceeds, the infant gathers enough of a self to recognize that he and another are different or separate

Tragic man – Kohut found that psychoanalysis needed to create meaning, in distinction to Freud who found that psychoanalysis needed to relieve the suffering of guilt

Twinning – another basic need of the baby to merge or be like powerful others

Twinship transference – Kohut's belief that some patients need to see themselves as "like" their analysts and therefore as positive

Vicarious introspection – the form of empathy Kohut believed would allow the patient to feel understood and valued

References

Beebe, B. & Lachmann, F.M. (2002) *Infant Research and Adult Treatment.* Hillsdale, NJ: Analytic Press.

Brandchaft, B., Doctors, S., & Sorter, D. (2010) *Towards an Emancipatory Psychoanalysis.* New York: Routledge.

Buber, M. (1958) *I and Thou.* New York: Scribner.

Ekman, P. (2003) *Emotions Revealed.* New York: Times Books.

Kohut, H. (1959) Introspection, empathy and psychoanalysis: An examination of the relationship between mode of observation and theory. In *The Search for the Self,* vol. 1. Madison, CT International Universities Press, 1978.

Kohut, H. (1971) *The Analysis of the Self.* New York: International Universities Press.
Kohut, H. (1972) Thoughts on narcissism and narcissistic rage. In *The Search for the Self,* vol 2. Madison, CT International Universities Press, 1978.
Kohut, H. (1977) *The Restoration of the Self.* New York: International Universities Press.
Kohut, H. (1984) *How Does Analysis Cure?* Chicago: University of Chicago Press.
Mitchell, S.A. (1993) *Hope and Dread in Psychoanalysis.* New York: Basic Books.
Mitchell, S.A. & Black, M. (1995) *Freud and Beyond.* New York: Basic Books.
Morrison, A.P. (1984) Shame and the psychology of the self. In Stepansky, P.E. & Goldberg, A. (eds) *Kohut's Legacy.* Hillsdale, NJ: Analytic Press.
Orange, D.M. (2010) *Thinking for Clinicians.* New York: Routledge.
Orange, D.M. (2011) *The Suffering Stranger.* New York: Routledge.
Ruesch, J. & Bateson, G. (1951) *Communication: The Social Matrix of Psychiatry.* New York: Norton.
Siegel, D.J. (2007) *The Mindful Brain.* New York: Norton.
Stern, D.N. (1985) *The Interpersonal World of the Infant.* New York: Basic Books.
Stern, D.N. (2004) *The Present Moment in Psychotherapy and Everyday Life.* New York: Norton.
Stolorow, R.D. (2007) *Trauma and Human Existence.* New York; Analytic Press.
Stolorow, R.D. & Atwood, G.E. (1992) *Contexts of Being: The Intersubjective Foundations of Psychological Life.* Hillsdale, NJ: Analytic Press.
Stolorow, R.D. & Lachman, F.M. (1980) *Psychoanalysis of Developmental Arrests.* Madison, CT: International Universities Press.
Strozier, C.B. (2001) *Heinz Kohut: The Making of a Psychoanalyst.* New York: Farrar, Straus & Giroux.

7

HARRY SULLIVAN

We need relationships to manage our anxieties and to thrive

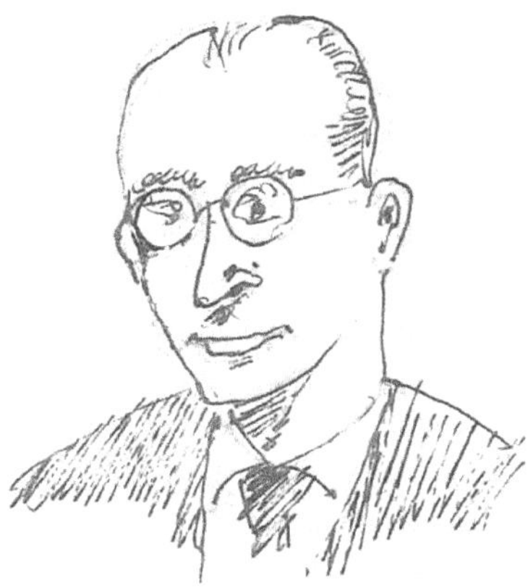

Harry Sullivan

American psychiatrist Harry S. Sullivan (1892–1949) was a key founder of the American interpersonal psychoanalytic school, often referred to as the relational school. His isolated childhood spent in upstate New York deeply informed his empathic understanding of isolation, anxiety, loneliness, and even poverty. He had a doting but unstable mother and experienced a psychotic break of his own while in college, further contributing to his insights about serious mental illness (Perry, 1982). He was a civilian doctor during World War I and then spent his professional life working in several hospitals along the East Coast and later in private practice in New York City and teaching in various institutions. He published little but taught a lot and interacted often with other important analysts, spreading his radical reformulation of Freud's ideas. Beginning in 1940, his lectures were consolidated and published, solidifying his extensive remaking of the analytic project.

As a young man, Sullivan struggled to find his own path, eventually settling on psychiatry. After World War I, he found an administrative job in a hospital in Washington DC under the leadership of the already well-known William Alanson White. White was extremely important to the brilliant yet socially awkward Sullivan, opening many doors to institutions and individuals as they shared many intellectual interests and dreams (Perry, 1982).

Sullivan immersed himself in his next job, working in a small unit of schizophrenics at Sheppard Pratt Hospital in Maryland. He held a deep interest in psychosis and he did not find the prevailing, exclusively biological theories of American psychiatry helpful. So, he turned to the Freudian talking cure, introduced to him by White.

Sullivan's experiences with his patients differed dramatically from Freud's experiences. Freud had found an unconscious, which must be uncovered and challenged, as it was full of unacceptable impulses and fantasies. In his patients, Sullivan found unbearable loneliness and a self-system designed to ward off anxiety. Almost immediately, he came to believe that life is lived inter-personally and that context is formative. He theorized that humans are always constructing themselves in the interpersonal moment and that the interpersonal world is the source of psychopathology, not the Freudian-based intra-psychic. For him, personality is only manifest in the interpersonal situation. He also acknowledged the impact of poverty on his patients. The unit of study became the interpersonal field, not the individual inside his skin (Sullivan, 1940; 1953).

It is hard to imagine today how radically both Sullivan's theory and technique broke new ground. In the 1920s there was only one form of psychotherapy and it was Freudian psychoanalysis, which was already known and established in the US. To be an analyst, you needed to have been in analysis. Analysis was for neurotics. The analytic stance was studied neutrality. Initially, Sullivan was an outsider, breaking all of these rules and conventions, inventing something totally new, thrilled to talk about it and teach it.

In order to relate first to the schizophrenics on his ward and later to other types of patients, he quickly changed his therapy format from the Freudian-based neutral listening with occasional interpretations to one of active questioning (Mitchell & Black, 1995). It is only with attention and questions that Sullivan can find out all the details—what is really going on with this person he is sitting with, what is the pattern that is being created, re-created? He advocated that the psychiatrist should continuously reflect internally on what the other is experiencing in the moment. "What is my best guess as to what he thinks I think of him?" Sullivan maintained that no matter what diagnosis the other carried, the psychiatrist knows subjectively something about that condition (Sullivan, 1940; 1970).

He became very interested in language itself and how we each use language in very different ways. He noted that seriously mentally ill people use language almost exclusively for defense—to protect themselves and their self-esteem—while others can afford to reveal more of themselves with safety. He believed that the only way to get to know and understand another is to have meaningful conversations using his probing questions. He sought to discover the tiniest details of what actually happened in the therapy session, whether reported from the past or in the present moment. For Sullivan, all of human life is to be found in this interpersonal space—the space between two human beings. His posthumous book, *The Psychiatric Interview*, is devoted to that continuous interest: How can we get to know another human being?—a very difficult project (Sullivan, 1970).

He was clear that we can't achieve it by staying objective and distant. His famous phrase was to become a "participant observer" (Sullivan, 1940). The analyst internally acknowledges his own reactions to the patient and uses this information to help him develop ideas about the patient's needs, fantasies, defenses. At the same time, the psychiatrist stays the expert, never drawn into enacting their own defenses and certainly never needing anything from the patient.

By the early 1920s, he had devised "milieu therapy" in hospital settings as the logical healing format emerging from his belief that the interpersonal space is key to both psychopathology and healing. For a time, he lived on the grounds of one of those hospitals and encouraged the staff to drop by and talk about what they were experiencing with their patients. Based on these conversations, he set up a ward for young male psychotics with an all-male staff, which had a particularly high success rate. They made what he called "social recoveries" (Perry, 1982). The practices he instituted continued to be successful under his successors.

In Sullivan's model, needs are what connect us, in contrast to Freud's position, that needs are problems to be solved. He referred to needs as integrating tendencies as they are what bring people together, creating reciprocal satisfaction throughout life (Mitchell & Black, 1995). His developmental model involves the infant moving between comfort and tension, always in the context of an "other." If the babe's needs are met, tension is reduced, and both the self and the relationship are safe and ongoing. The infant legitimately needs his significant other (Sullivan, 1940). This need for others continues throughout all the developmental stages and, when these needs are not met appropriately, intense loneliness and/or various forms of pathology develop.

These needs for connection and satisfaction are inherent. If these needs are not met, tension increases and turns into anxiety which is not inherent. In his interesting use of language, the feeling of fear itself is an integrating tendency as when expressed it brings the carer closer. Anxiety is not the inherent fear that connects. Rather anxiety comes from others and constitutes the basic disintegrating impulse. I believe that because of his own history, Sullivan had an interesting twist in his basic formulation around anxiety. He proposed that anxiety in the child derives from anxiety in the caregiver rather than the baby creating and experiencing his own anxiety directly. Like others, he realized that this makes anxiety impossible to resolve because the source of the baby's anxiety is in fact an anxious parent, who should have been the baby's comforter. The baby has an unsolvable dilemma when both the needed potential soother and the source of anxiety reside in the same external other. Sullivan held that anxious and non-anxious are the keys to a "bad" or a "good" mother. He coined the phrase "selective inattention," the process by which the child ignores the mother's anxiety in order to avoid feeling anxious himself (Mitchell & Black, 1995).

In Sullivan's (1940; 1953) model, the self is created over time through interactions with the environment. The baby slowly learns to read the approaching other, who is beyond his control. However, later, the young child realizes that some of his behaviors affect the other, both positively and negatively. The behaviors that elicit warmth from outside gradually become the "good me." When anxiety is in the field, the child experiences his own version of "bad me."

His healthy self-system is conservative but not rigid or fixed. If there has been too much anxiety, the self-system will be too rigid and new experiences cannot be used for learning and growth (Sullivan, 1940).

Sullivan distinguished a hierarchy of needs which he labeled the need for security and the need for satisfaction (Mitchell & Black, 1995). Safety and security are not part of the classical formulations; these are new concerns requiring new techniques. Only when security needs are met can the individual reach out for true satisfaction. We might say this is the difference between surviving and thriving. Interpersonal analysts in the Sullivan lineage ask many questions, wanting to formulate the best questions for self-discovery. Eventually, a question will alert the anxiety-managing system so it can be faced, understood, and soothed. They keep their focus mostly on here-and-now issues, the current life issues of the patient and the experiences of the patient with the analyst. This is in contrast to the intersubjective analysts, who are more likely to keep their developmental model in mind and look for the developmental arrests that keep creativity and joy at bay.

After his intense period of living and working on hospital grounds, Sullivan moved to New York City to open a private practice, to teach up and down the East Coast, and to exchange ideas with both colleagues and artists. In the 1930s, he and several others established the William Alanson White Psychiatric Foundation along with the *American Journal of Psychiatry*. Both eventually became leading intellectual centers of psychoanalysis in America and laid the foundation for what became the relational school.

In the years that followed, during World War II, Sullivan served on the American Psychiatric Association's committee on military mobilization. Through the use of psychiatric screening, he both wanted to create a fine military and avoid stigmatizing the men who were unfit for military service but very fit for life in other ways. This was a difficult balance to achieve and he and others struggled with it throughout the war. After the war, he was committed to helping set up institutions that would further peace in the world. In spite of knowing he had a serious heart condition, he set out for Paris in 1949 for a United Nations Educational, Scientific and Cultural Organization meeting and died while on his way to France (Perry, 1982).

Sullivan always considered his interpersonal theory a school of psychiatry, not limited to psychoanalysis (Mitchell & Black, 1995). He thought along a continuum from fleeting anxiety to severe pathology and taught that a phenomenological investigation of self was the key to understanding the other (Sullivan, 1953). Over time, he generated a complete alternative to Freud's drive theory, observing the same human issues through a very different lens: the body, sexuality, pleasure, aggression, and constitution, even the concept of the "good life." His followers have developed a true, two-person theory of personality, psychopathology, and healing. The rest of this chapter is devoted to some of those analytic followers and their thoughts that I have found most useful. The school itself is very large and diverse, although its members do all share a common interest in the interpersonal as the domain of study for both pathology and healing. The relational school maintains that the contents of the intrapsychic life were formed by the internalization of interpersonal experiences rather than drives meeting reality.

ERICH FROMM

Erich Fromm (1900–1980) made major theoretical contributions to humanistic psychology, political psychology, and social psychology, and strongly influenced the relational school. For a time in the 1920s, in Germany, he became a traditional psychoanalyst, opening his own practice in 1927. However, like many others, Fromm had to flee Nazi Germany, first for Switzerland, and then for America. He met Sullivan in the 1930s and was one of the founders of the White Institute. He taught, wrote about, and practiced psychoanalysis in the US and Mexico for the rest of his professional life. His books have been popular both within analytic circles and with thoughtful people in the wider population. His small book, *The Art of Loving*, has been enjoyed by millions and translated into many languages. For Fromm, love is an interpersonal, creative act that requires effort and will. It is not an emotion; rather, it combines care, responsibility, respect, and knowledge of the other. He believed that we dread isolation and loneliness more than anything else and that the antidote to this dread is a loving connection. His conversation with Freud was one of open disagreement around many issues including love, our need for connection and sexuality (Fromm, 1956).

His first book in 1941, which is still popular today, was *Escape from Freedom*. For Fromm, freedom or free will is always available; we either embrace it or deny it. In his way of experiencing life, when we deny our capacity for freedom, we enter a world of conflict and blame. We lie to ourselves and to each other, valuing conformity over autonomy. He outlined different aspects of possible avoidance of personal responsibility: "Automaton conformity" requires me to change my true self into an ideal more favored by my society. Then, I am no longer responsible for my actions and myself; instead, society is responsible for me and makes my choices for me. If I engage in an "authoritarian relationship" with the world, I give over my capacity to make choices to others (Fromm, 1941).

He argued that each of us needs to find our place in the world, where we fit or belong. Ideally, we are given our first security with our mother, but it is our task to grow beyond that kind of security and find our home in the wider world. He was very critical of social conditions that do not foster these necessary connections.

His model for meaning and the good life involved this sense of freedom and choice. He recommended that we choose to actively love and work in the world, thwarting alienation and isolation.

For Fromm, the unconscious is a "social creation" like the rest of our sense of self, which is formed within our primary relationships and then sustained by what he termed our "fear of freedom." If we are to express our authentic self, we risk isolation. In his work, he exhorted each of us to hold the tension between connection and individuation, creating our unique way in the world (Fromm, 1947).

Fromm influenced the relational school in two very important ways (Mitchell & Black, 1995). He strongly emphasized working in the present and keeping the focus of the analytic hour on how the patient was living in the present. Second, he wrote that analytic neutrality was artificial contributing to inauthentic living. Even Sullivan's participant observer was too distant for Fromm.

Because of his belief in authenticity, he writes that the analyst, the humanistic analyst, must respond honestly and frankly to his patients, providing an antidote to the chronic dishonesty of society (Mitchell & Black, 1995). His focus was neither on developmental issues nor conflict issues. Rather, he focused on loneliness, the need for connection, and the need for freedom in order not to feel trapped by life and its responsibilities. He is wonderful to read and think about; however, much of Fromm's writing is beyond the scope of this book, as it is directed toward collective, political, and religious life.

I often think of Fromm's emphasis on freedom and loneliness when sitting with Jess. She and her husband are retired, her children are grown and married, her mother is well cared for. Yet Jess speaks of being trapped, first by her own style of thinking and speaking slowly and then by the demands of her family. She feels lonely much of the time in spite of being surrounded by people who love her. Once she has found her words in my office, I am genuinely involved in what she personally needs, feels, and wants, creating the longed-for connection. She has discovered that she needs more one-on-one time, that life within the three-generational family is tumultuous and fun, but not nourishing to her personal way of being. She has begun to carve out time with individual family members and girlfriends to meet her personal need for deeper connection. This has been surprisingly hard for her, as her old way of being was solely based on meeting the needs of others. As Fromm wrote, the effort required has been great and the fear of losing connection by asking for what she wants has been intense.

CLARA THOMPSON

Clara Thompson (1893–1958) was yet another American psychiatrist and psychoanalyst who made important contributions to the relational tradition, including the creation of the White Institute. She was academically brilliant and initially intended to become a medical missionary. Over time, she gave up her interest in religion and focused first on medicine and then on psychoanalysis. She opened her own practice in 1925 and, in 1931, moved to Budapest to undergo a full analysis with the both controversial and beloved Sándor Ferenczi. She was in treatment with him until his death in 1933 (Moulton, 1986).

Upon her return to the US, she combined the work of her American colleagues and friends—especially Sullivan and Fromm—with that of Ferenczi, changing the focus of her analytic work from the past to the present. Like others, she broke with Freud over what she felt was the reality of child abuse, as opposed to the imagined internal relational dynamics Freud proposed. As a teacher, Thompson was well-versed in all current branches of psychoanalysis, seemingly respecting them, all the while contending that psychoanalysis needed to evolve in order to reach more people and help everyone become more human (Thompson, 1950).

Thompson was among the first psychoanalytic thinkers to focus on the differences between men and women, and she wrote many papers on the psychology of women (Moulton, 1986). She noted how our society and culture were changing the roles available to women and the conflicts that are inherent in such role changes. The journey from self-sacrificing mother and wife to wanting a profession and seeking fulfillment outside the home is long and complex. She strongly criticized Freud's bias against women as inherently inferior and wrote about women's sexuality in a much more positive light. This is not the place to expand on this first wave of feminism, but Thompson and many of her colleagues helped normalize a psychology of women that is different from but in no way inferior to the psychology of men.

Like Sullivan, Thompson's view of the therapeutic dyad was one of "participant observer." The role of the analyst is to stay slightly outside of the interaction while participating fully with care and intellectual curiosity: "What is going on here between us? What would make the patient feel safer? What triggered the present emotion?" For her, the relationship between patient and therapist was the key, as the current relationship embodies all the salient aspects of formative past relationships. Deep and genuine caring is key to healing, as this is what determines whether or not the patient will feel safe enough to explore internally and then reveal what is deeply troubling them (Thompson, 1950).

Let's return to Jess. Her old way was to put everyone else first, often not knowing what she desired. Now in retirement, she finds a good outer life but chronic loneliness on the inside. I see this as a typically female pattern of relating, which has good and loving aspects. At birth, babies need to be put first, and children need care for many years if they are to thrive. Jess has discovered the truth of what Thompson wrote about decades ago. Women need more in their lives than the project of raising children and tending the home. Self-expression and intimacy are what Jess needs and, through our work together, she is finding both.

The changing role of the analyst

In contemporary relational psychoanalysis, the analyst is no longer Sullivan's or Thompson's participant observer, paying attention to both but slightly outside of the dyad. Now there are two co-participants, each contributing to the interactive events in the consulting room. Contemporary relational analysts assume they have needs and anxieties as well as their own security operations or defenses (Aron, 1990). We have arrived at a fully two-person system in that both participants co-create what is happening. The analyst monitors their responses to the situation internally and uses those emotional responses as data relevant to the conversation. Furthermore, the contemporary relational analyst holds that the patient's beliefs about the analyst are based on lived experience; they are not merely products from the patient's past and his imagination. Things happen in the context of a therapy session that are crucial for both parties (Aron, 1991, 1996).

For this analyst, neutrality is no longer possible. They are neither a blank screen, nor a reflecting mirror. This analyst assumes that the dynamics between the two parties will create what are called enactments. Instead of an exclusive focus on the patient's acting out—that is, breaking the frame or resisting the basic injunction—enactments acknowledge the analyst's equal capacity to act out, to allow his real self and his real reactions to influence his role. Currently, it is believed that, together, the salient interpersonal dynamics of the patient's life will be recreated and lived through the dyadic relationship. Ideally, the analyst will become aware of the re-enactment and be able to think about it, reflect on it, point out the patient's part in it, and crucially own their own contributions. Again, this is the ideal and often not the reality. The simple truth is there are two imperfect humans in the room. Nevertheless, much growth can come of this.

Over the years, I have worked with several women who have left abusive relationships. They carry the scars of both physical and emotional abuse—an inner frozenness and an inability to learn new ways of relating and to trust that things could be different between two adults. At some point in each therapy, I have inadvertently expressed my impatience with these women in a minor but significant way, perhaps by verbally chastising them about a repetitive pattern. They have never complained about my choice of words or tone. This represents a clear enactment on both our parts. In a titrated way, I have become the abuser to their victim. Each time, I must catch myself, apologize, and help them express how awful it felt to be chastised by the person who is supposed to be on their side. This is made doubly delicate by their automatic compliance. Internally, I first wonder and then speak: Does it feel bad to be chastised, or are you complying with my suggestion that it must feel bad? How do we discern the difference?

This dramatically different analytic position has its own set of problems. We will touch on some of them as we delve further into the tradition discussing Lewis Aron, Stephen Mitchell, and Philip Bromberg.

LEWIS ARON

Contemporary American Lewis Aron has been a major figure in the relational tradition since the early 1990s, as the editor of *Psychoanalytic Dialogues*, the author of several books, and the co-editor with Stephen Mitchell of the giant *Relational Psychoanalysis*. He first came to my attention with his article on one-person and two-person psychology (Aron, 1990). In that article, he writes of how classical analysis is strictly one-person and why that stance is not truly helpful to the patient. Using the mother–child analogy, he notes that the mother is real, has her own inner life, and that she is not only a baby minder. The growing infant gets to know his mother intimately as a person. According to Aron, the patient needs to know the essence of his analyst—that is, he needs to know his analyst as a person in order for analysis to be curative. For Aron and all the relational analysts, two-person psychology is required, not an opaque, blank screen.

Along those same lines, he emphasizes examining the patient's direct experience of the analyst, not through interpretation but through a more open-ended inquiry. All analytic relationships are asymmetrical in both role and responsibility despite even a two-person stance. The analyst must responsibly ask what they believe to be the best reflective questions to further the treatment. We can imagine Sullivan and Thompson would be asking questions about the patient's life and relationships. While those questions would still be presented, the bigger focus for Aron (1991) would be on the immediate relationship and the feelings of the moment. It is very different to ask, "What did you think about me when I said that?" than to ask, "What happened inside when you said that to your boss?"

Freud and his contemporaries envisioned the mind as existing inside the head of each participant as an autonomous and independent actor. For Aron, the relational school, and most modern therapists, the mind is inherently dyadic, social, interactional, and interpersonal. From this perspective, to investigate the mind of another is to investigate the intersubjective field, somewhat like the self psychologists. Many of the differences between the self psychologists and the relational psychologists are clarified in the following section on Stephen Mitchell.

Aron advocates consistent attention to the co-creation of the meanings generated by the patient and analyst. Together, these form a system, each affecting the other moment by moment. Aron's context is very much the "here and now," not the "there and then" of the Freudian archeology. This brings a very different sensibility to the therapeutic process.

In Aron and Starr's *A Psychotherapy for the People* (2013), they once again start the conversation with a Freud quote, noting that Freud wanted analysis to be widely available to help everyone. The book is a fascinating, intimate history of psychoanalytic ideas, but the concept that has most helped me is that of "mutual vulnerability." In his earlier work, Aron has always talked about a whole range of mutualities—from influence to empathy. But here is a new one: the analyst's need to be what they call "permeable, mortal, human." They write that mutual vulnerability leads to transformed and spiritualized healing. For me, it is as if the austere stereotype of classical analysis has morphed into a very humanistic stance without sacrificing any of its intellectual rigor. We are light and dark, conscious and unconscious, and all of each of us is truly available in the present moment if we can deeply listen and pay attention.

I often use Aron's focus on the present moment when I sit with Dan. His emotions have seemingly dried up and no longer fuel any conscious desires. Dan's aridity inhibits every aspect of expression verbal and non-verbal. He offers little about his external life, thus forcing the conversation into the room and the space between us. At first, Dan was nonplussed when I asked him about the fantasies he had while driving to my office, what crossed his mind when he thought about talking to me on a given day. Lately, he is a little more comfortable with this way of participating in our relationship as we explore what happens between us. We wonder together about what is helpful and not helpful in furthering his desire for more connection in the outer world by noticing how we are connected and not connected.

STEPHEN MITCHELL

It is fair to say that the American Stephen Mitchell (1946–2000) was among the most influential of the interpersonal or relational analysts, and it is tragic that his contributions ended in 2000 with his untimely death. Mitchell has written extensively linking theory and technique of relational psychoanalysis with every other school and he has deeply influenced my way of practicing. In his many publications, he addresses everyone from Freud to Kohut, to Winnicott and Sullivan (Mitchell & Black, 1995). That makes him an extremely valuable resource for any clinical or theoretical exploration. I would categorize him as a both/and kind of thinker, as he finds value in many ideas and approaches. However, he clearly privileges relational theory over drive theory (Aron & Starr, 2013). He respectfully lays out a thinker's position on a given issue and then makes a case for why a more interpersonal or relational approach is better. This approach creates a space for each clinician to find their own way concerning that issue. For Mitchell, the basic unit of study was not the individual as a separate entity, but the interactional field between a person and their significant others both past and present and between each patient and analyst. This process is continual and ongoing as each struggles to make contact and be understood. In his model, desire is always experienced within the context of a relationship, and each relationship creates its own meaning. For Mitchell, the mind is composed of these relational configurations. Analysis relieves suffering by attending to what is happening in the present between analyst and patient, not past history or attention to developmental issues (Mitchell, 1993).

Unlike both the middle school and the self psychologists, for Mitchell (1993), the analyst is not a mirror, not devoted exclusively to attuning to the patient. Instead, the analyst is a meaning-making subjectivity in his own right, meeting another meaning-making subjectivity. The questions become how do we both deal with this reality, the reality that there are two of us here, sitting here, struggling together here. What does the analyst know? What does the patient need?

Mitchell has written extensively on the evolution of psychoanalysis, demonstrating his profound understanding of the various schools of thought, the individual thinkers, and their relationships to specific concepts (Mitchell & Black, 1995). He loved thinking and psychoanalysis, and he cared deeply for those who came to him. He wrote of his own responses to his patients in a true two-person fashion, honoring his own stance that each relationship is unique (Mitchell, 1993). He knew what he had to offer his patients: that, through treatment, they will enlarge and enrich themselves; that they will have more access to their memories; that they will have a better sense of their unique complexity; that they will be more future-oriented; and, most importantly, that they will have a stronger sense of agency, along with the capacity to affect their personal future. People enter analysis because they are suffering in some way—perhaps they are victims of outer circumstances ("My husband left me out of the blue") or inner unconscious, usually self-destructive impulses ("I don't know what happened; I just had to get out of there"). For Mitchell, success does not mean suffering ends; rather, it means his patients know themselves to be the creators of their lives within the limits of their circumstances. It means they have become the author of their own lives (Mitchell, 1997).

Developmental tilt and the emphasis on conflict

Staying focused in the present helps to avoid what Mitchell called "developmental tilt," which means too much emphasis on early formative years, suggesting the patient is frozen in the past (Mitchell, 1988). Mitchell was addressing Kohut's developmental arrest model, which is the basis of the self-psychology lineage as well as object-relations theorists with their strong theoretical interest in the first years of life. Mitchell believed that the self-psychology analysts offer to gratify the intense needs of the baby with empathic immersion rather than confronting and integrating those needs. Mitchell insists that we talk about those needs and desires, sorting them into what is appropriate for the adult and what represents the past with its intense anxiety.

Like Fairbairn, Mitchell wrote that theory and practice must align. He worried that, with too much emphasis on developmental arrest, there would be a tendency to coddle and infantilize rather than robustly address presently occurring conflicts in the therapeutic relationship. Mitchell wanted conflict and disagreement out in the open in order for the patient to be seen as an adult and—eventually—to see himself as an adult. For Mitchell and the relational school, the patient is always an active participant in the interaction, never a helpless child caught in developmental arrest.

In each relationship, the patient and the analyst re-create their known and unknown conflicts—in part to re-create the familiar, in part to enter unknown territory that needs to be explored, and in part to find safety. Both participate in this need to recreate. Both are on their "edge," in the context of necessary safety (Mitchell, 1988; 1993).

At times, Mitchell referred to the relational model as the relational-conflict model. When the patient enters therapy, he wants something new while also wanting to hold on to the old and familiar. From the start, he will engage the therapist from his habitual ways of being. The analyst must respond authentically, continually discovering and revealing himself within the relationship and sharing what he finds in a way that the patient can use for his own growth. For Mitchell, therapy is collaboration, for both parties must engage in the effort to understand what is being created in the present moment. The analyst must commit himself fully to the relationship, expressing his care and his frustrations. These are the hallmarks of true engagement and authentic moment-to-moment connection (Mitchell, 1997).

Working in the present

The relational model privileges the interaction within the present moment. During each hour, both therapist and patient are struggling to maintain key tensions: autonomy and connection, individuation and attachment, self and other regulation, and the management of subjective and objective reality. Like Erikson, Mitchell believed development continues throughout the life cycle and that each new encounter is a new opportunity for hope and change rather than the deadness of repetition. For him, earliest experiences are meaningful not because they lay down fixed structural residues, but because they are the earliest representations of patterns that will be repeated over and over again (Mitchell, 1988). Understanding the past is important, not because the past is hidden under the present, but because the past provides clues that are helpful in deciphering why the present is approached in this particular way. Mitchell acknowledged the need for adult interdependence. He found that most patients have foreclosed direct and appropriate adult negotiations, leaving them bereft of the kind of connections that further healthy interdependence.

I appreciate Mitchell's (1993) writing on hope as I believe it is foundational to the human experience. He notes that psychoanalysis has had two very different approaches to hope: regressive and progressive. In the Freudian tradition, hope has been seen as a mix of infantile fantasy and illusion. This kind of hope wishes for easy and early gratifications. For Freud and his followers, it is the renunciation of illusions and the acknowledgment of reality that informs maturity.

The other side of hope is the genuine hope of a new beginning, the connection to authentic living and real desire. Mitchell suggests this side of the hope story is clearly laid out by Erikson and his notion of basic trust—his source of hope throughout life. For Erikson, hope is always growth-inducing. Winnicott also believed in hope, especially in his writings about delinquents, naming their actions as based on hope, hope that their needs could finally be met. (See sidebar in Chapter 8.) Kohut and Bromberg are other examples of analysts who see hope in their patients' demands.

Atypically, Mitchell also writes of the analyst's hopes: their desire to help the other, to create meaning for their own lives through this endeavor. Therapists and analysts alike have a lot invested in seeing the other grow and change. Is that not hope?

I know that I begin every therapy with the hope that I can be helpful to the suffering of the other. When I am challenged, I read more, I find the appropriate supervision. Each of the people I have presented has challenged me in specific ways and I always hope that I have helped in some way—helped uncover a more authentic self, helped re-start some frozen aspect of being.

PHILIP BROMBERG

Philip Bromberg is another contemporary American who has greatly enhanced our understanding of early childhood relational trauma. He writes in both the traditional analytic language (Bromberg, 2006) and the newer language of trauma, including the terms "affect regulation" and "dysregulation" (Bromberg, 1998; 2011). He is deeply interested in dissociation, both normal and pathological. He uses literature, movies, and neuroscience to enhance his ideas, which makes reading him especially pleasurable (2006; 2011). His developmental model describes the child needing total regulation from the parents at the beginning of life. Within the first year and beyond,this capacity needs to slowly be taken over by the individual himself. When there is too much trauma at the beginning of life, the individual has not accumulated the resources to take care of their emotional "ongoingness." This is now spoken of as "developmental trauma" and is a very different idea from the Freudian notion of drives and conflicts (Bromberg, 2011). Children must have their subjective states both mirrored and attended to in a timely manner by others in order to feel good and real and whole. If this does not happen enough, the child cannot bear—let alone integrate—all of their good and bad feelings as part of a fluid "me." Bromberg notes that dissociation is always available and is a normal response when emotional life becomes unbearable. With too much trauma, our capacity to dissociate becomes an internal structure rather than an option. Dissociation narrows and limits the patient's life, creating a self-protective, constrained self-state. Such an individual typically becomes hyper-vigilant, always waiting for and looking for bad things to happen.

Dissociation

One of the original Freudian defenses, dissociation is now considered the hallmark of trauma, whether it is relational trauma or the force of an external event, such as a natural disaster, rape, or war. The term refers to splits within the psyche or within awareness, where parts of the self are absolutely not known to other parts of the self. These missing parts are not repressed — put out of awareness by guilt as in the Freudian understanding — rather, they are so utterly unbearable that they cannot be experienced without overwhelming the psyche. Therefore, they are split off and frozen before they ever reach awareness.

Safe surprise

Bromberg teaches us that these developmentally traumatized patients live in a state of constant danger, terror, shame, and vigilance. He advises that the therapeutic relationship must become a place that simultaneously offers safety while supporting risk taking (Bromberg, 2006; 2011). In each specific therapeutic relationship, the pain of early trauma must be experienced in a titrated form without the consequences of increased dissociation and hidden pain, the old experience. In the present safe therapeutic context, the upset is allowed, not stopped or shamed. It is important to put words on the experience, understand what is happening, and through this understanding transform the affective upset from a life-threatening danger to something smaller and more manageable. Bromberg calls this "safe but not too safe" or the "safe surprise." It is up to the analyst to keep the patient emotionally safe and, at the same time, keep the therapy on the edge of growth.

Bromberg has augmented the analytic conversation itself through the personal quality of his professional writings. In most instances, he keeps very much to the topic at hand, writing in a third-person format in very formal language. But, occasionally, he allows us into his personal history and his private thoughts, sharing his associations, where he limits himself, and where he feels free to "play" (Bromberg, 2011).

In the chapter on Kohut, I mentioned how often I failed Jack and how necessary it is for us to navigate multiple ruptures and repairs. Jack lives in the world of developmental trauma: the emotional world of rage and terror that Bromberg so eloquently describes. Through my questions and his associations, it has become clear that Jack dissociates from the feelings of his early life while remembering the facts clearly. He has always subjectively felt in danger, from earliest childhood until today. For Jack, the two biggest dangers are being abandoned and being shamed. He seldom speaks directly, preferring to speak in metaphors. One of his favorites is that of "war." When he is at war, which is most of the time, his real feelings don't matter. They are, in fact, both irrelevant and a nuisance. What matters is achieving the goal, either personally or professionally. Jack can carry this off when things go well, but when he meets obstacles, he falls into what he calls a "state." At home, when he is in such a state, he wants to watch TV with his wife at his side. He can't bear being alone but also can't bear conversation or interaction of any kind. In my office, it has become clear that this state is pure terror. Underneath the state of dissociation which holds him together, he is utterly dysregulated. In my office, when we can get under that states he falls into extreme agony, shaking and crying. When we can be together for these times, I observe that it moves through him in huge waves, eventually subsiding into the relief of survival. Nowhere else does he feel safe enough to allow the feeling of terror to fully exist.

Self-states

Bromberg has changed the theoretical conversation completely by introducing the concept of "self-states." He delineates both what he refers to as the normal, multiple selves of all human beings and those aspects of traumatized people that appear and disappear with no inner continuity (Bromberg, 1998). For him, the ego is not managing an id, nor are there objects and part objects or selfobjects. Rather, Bromberg (2011) states clearly there is no one self, no singular, true, authentic self. Instead, we live among our multiple self-states, ideally flowing from one to the other without undue stress. This would be authentic, creative living, another way of conceptualizing a true self. However, with developmental trauma, these inner states are unknown one to the other. Jack exemplifies this every time he is stressed. The high-functioning businessman disappears—one self-state—and the terrified, shameful aspect of himself appears as his entire sense of self. In that moment, he is only shame and terror. Both are real and, in that sense, both are true. But they are not creative or playful. They are rigid and fixed, bound and controlled by a context, rather than coming from agency and spontaneity.

I find Bromberg's (2011) notion of the complexity of truth in analysis helpful, even hopeful and reassuring. He notes over and over that we try and fail. That uncertainty surrounds the dyad. That conflict and surprise are signs of aliveness. We are always two subjects sitting together wanting to understand each other, wanting to create relational intimacy, and wanting to evolve into greater wholeness. Each needs the other and both are fundamentally equal in Buber's (1958) I–thou sense, in spite of the asymmetry of the relationship.

The impact on therapy/analysis of the changing frame: personal reflections

In the classical model, the analyst is an authority and all transactions—ranging from the most mundane to the most psychologically important—are assumed to originate from within the patient. However, aspects of the frame are fixed by the analyst. For example, historically each patient "owns" certain hours of the week and if he does not use those hours, he still pays for them. The metaphor of the parking garage is often employed: You own the spot whether you use it or not. This kind of certainty is seldom possible today, as clients demand much more flexibility, yet the analyst also must have their own needs met, regarding both time and money.

Currently, cancellations and changes to session times have become the norm, and each therapist has to come to their own way of dealing with such issues. Is there a general policy? Are decisions made on a case-by-case basis? What about extenuating circumstances? Modern therapists, who see the relationship as a significant part of healing, struggle to find their place along the continuum outlined by the relational school. Some lean toward the participant-observer style of Sullivan and Thompson. Others are inclined toward the fuller engagement proposed by

Aron, Mitchell, and Bromberg. I find that both have their place in a long-term therapy. Language and words matter significantly. For example, I may struggle with a new client who wants a particular time of day—a time I have available only once a week. When his work interferes, he wants to come another day that week at that same time and I do not have availability at his preferred time. I can say either, "I am sorry that I have so little flexibility," or I can say, "I simply don't have another opening at your preferred time." I may or may not add, "I wish I did, but I don't." Each of these approaches conveys something slightly different and will have a different impact. The first takes the responsibility onto myself. The second pushes it toward him. With the last set of words, I am most clearly in my participant-observer mode, acknowledging that we have a problem and I can't solve it. I want to convey, "There is nothing wrong with your request, but we need to find a different time if we are to meet this week, and I hope we can."

Alternatively, I can widen the focus by saying, "I wonder why only this time is possible?" or, "I wish we each had more flexibility." With these words, I am more in my relational-conflict mode. The impact is different, even if it is not consciously registered. A number of questions arise: Do I wish to open a dialogue about his need for my schedule to be flexible while his is not? What are the constraints on his time, and how much are outer reality and how much are a very controlling "be perfect" inner voice leading to a rigid way of engaging the world? Is compliance to a spouse involved? Is he self-aware enough to be available for these kinds of dialogues or is that still to come down the road for us?

Therapists must always keep the relationship alive, real, and reflective of the lived experience of the moment. At the same time, our personal frustrations and needs as therapists can be damaging to the patient. Part of the art of good therapy is learning how to titrate our personal reactions with the need to stay authentic to the situation. Of course, we often fail this inner negotiation and when we do, an enactment follows. Hopefully that can be brought into awareness and repaired. If we can't repair it, usually the other will leave, as both the needs for safety and for being seen have been violated.

Like any therapist who has been in practice for decades, I have a long list of failed professional relationships. When I reflect on a failed relationship or a disappearance, either with my internal supervisor or with a colleague, I hypothesize a number of different possibilities. In hindsight, I might come to believe I over-accommodated in some situations—for example, lowering my fee until I became resentful, or working on weekends when it really wasn't convenient, or staying on the phone too long when I was too tired. Sometimes my own unconscious reacted in inappropriate ways—for example, laughing at something that was painful or becoming overtly annoyed at a too-often repeated story line. In an effort to be authentic I might have revealed something that upon reflection might be shaming to the other. Other times, I am surprised by a client's disappearance and simply never know what happened. I am always saddened, and at times disheartened, when I feel I have been unable to help.

Key concepts Chapter 8

Active questioning – Sullivan's technique to understand and help heal his patients; in distinction to the classical "blank screen" analyst

Affect regulation – refers to the universal need to manage both feelings and thoughts to maintain inner continuity

Developmental or strain trauma – when a parent does not meet a baby's needs in a timely and appropriate fashion the infant suffers; when this happens a lot, the infant's very sense of self is formed around the sense of not being taken care of, thus traumatized

Developmental tilt – Mitchell's stance that too often analysis privileges early childhood history over present-day interactions to the detriment of self-responsibility and growth

Dysregulation – refers to the human capacity to feel not whole, integrated, or good when thoughts and feelings run out of control; usually need another to regulate and provide safety and soothing

Enactments – inevitable behaviors that take place between analyst and patient that are created by unconscious frozen patterns that need to be "translated" into words and insight

Fear of freedom – Fromm's position that we fear fully being ourselves and instead comply to the wishes and demands of others in order to keep their love and connection

Interpersonal space – Sullivan's focus for treatment, less inside the other and more in the space between two living human beings

Intersubjective field – a further development of self psychology that conceives of the analytic relationship as composed of the space between two subjects working together on behalf of the patient

Milieu therapy – using inpatient settings Sullivan created a healing environment involving every aspect of living

Participant observation – an analytic stance that acknowledges the analyst's contribution to the relationship; at the same time the analyst and patient are not equals, the analyst keeps an appropriate distance monitoring the transaction

Relational-conflict model – Mitchell's understanding that the patient needs both a new relationship and a willingness to be confronted in difficult ways

Safe surprise – Bromberg's phrase for the best way to bring a new and perhaps challenging idea or insight into a patient's awareness

Selective inattention – Sullivan's phrase for how a child separates himself from his mother's anxiety

Self-states – Bromberg's acknowledgment that within each of us reside many different "selves," and sometimes these inner states are not overlapping or aware of each other

Significant other – Sullivan's observation that we need special people in our lives, starting with our first caregiver

References

Aron, L. (1990) One person and two person psychologies and the method of psychoanalysis. *Psychoanalytic Psychology*, 7: 475–485.
Aron, L. (1991) The patient's experience of the analyst's subjectivity. In Mitchell, S.A. & Aron, L. (eds) (1999) *Relational Psychoanalysis*. Hillsdale, NJ: Analytic Press.
Aron, L. (1996) *Meeting of Minds*. Hillsdale, NJ: Analytic Press.
Aron, L. & Starr, K. (2013) *A Psychotherapy for the People*. New York: Routledge.
Bromberg, P.M. (1998) *Standing in the Spaces*. Hillsdale, NJ: Analytic Press.
Bromberg, P.M. (2006) *Awakening the Dreamer*. Mahwah, NJ: Analytic Press.
Bromberg, P.M. (2011) *The Shadow of the Tsunami*. New York: Routledge.
Buber, M. (1958) *I and Thou*. New York: Charles Scribner's Sons.
Fromm, E. (1941) *Escape from Freedom*. New York: Avon.
Fromm, E. (1947) *Man for Himself*. Greenwich, CT: Fawcett.
Fromm, E. (1956) *The Art of Loving*. New York: Harper & Row.
Mitchell, S.A. (1988) *Relational Concepts in Psychoanalysis*. Boston, MA: Harvard.
Mitchell, S.A. (1993) *Hope and Dread in Psychoanalysis*. New York: Basic Books.
Mitchell, S.A. (1997) *Influence and Autonomy in Psychoanalysis*. Hillsdale, NJ: Analytic Press.
Mitchell, S. & Black, M. (1995) *Freud and Beyond*. New York: Basic Books.
Moulton, R. (1986) Clara Thompson: Unassuming leader. In Dickstein, L. & Nadelson, C. (eds) *Women Physicians in Leadership Roles*. Washington, DC: American Psychiatric Press.
Perry, H.S. (1982) *Psychiatrist of America: The Life of Harry Stack Sullivan*. Cambridge, MA: Harvard University Press.
Sullivan, H.S. (1940) *Conceptions of Modern Psychiatry*. New York: Norton.
Sullivan, H.S. (1953) *The Interpersonal Theory of Psychiatry*. New York: Norton.
Sullivan, H.S. (1970) *The Psychiatric Interview*. New York: Norton.
Thompson, C.M. (1950) *Psychoanalysis: Evolution and Development*. New York: Thomas Nelson.

8

JOHN BOWLBY

Lost connection is traumatic; secure attachment is the key to well-being

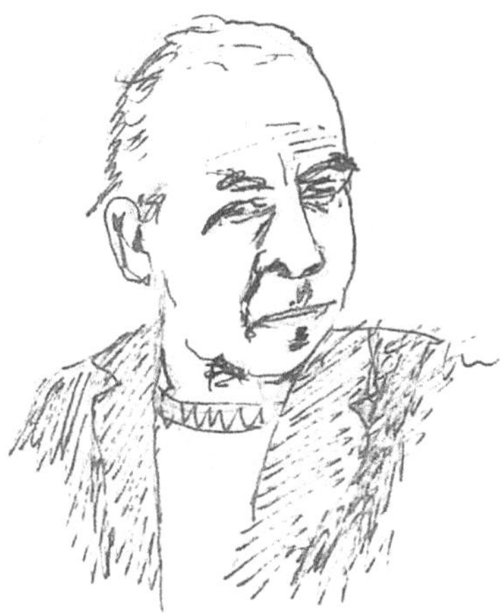

John Bowlby

Although all three branches of the British psychoanalytic community shunned him, John Bowlby (1907–1990) is a key figure in today's world of psychotherapy and psychoanalysis. He was rejected as being far too biological, mechanistic, and even simplistic in his thinking. He was criticized as reducing the human panoply of emotions and unconscious strivings—the whole Freudian project—into a single issue. His interest in ethnology had encouraged him to place human beings squarely in the world of mammals, who have basic needs, including a caregiver and, what he would call, attachment to that caregiver (Fonagy, 2001).

Bowlby was very much a product of the British upper class; he was raised by nannies with little contact with his parents, who believed that giving attention to a child would spoil or weaken him. He was sent to boarding school at age seven, which he hated. He later wrote that he was traumatized by these harsh and lonely experiences. However, he did survive and indeed thrive, eventually attending Cambridge, earning a medical degree, becoming a psychoanalyst, and, in due course, serving in World War II. After the war, he became the head of the Tavistock Clinic in London and a consultant to the World Health Organization (Bretherton, 1995; Holmes, 1995). In 1951, he published *Maternal Care and Mental Health*, in which he advocated that all infants need a warm, intimate, and continuous relationship with a mother or maternal substitute for at least two years. Bowlby devoted his life with unwavering focus to the infant's need for a secure early attachment. Through his research, he demonstrated that physical proximity to a caregiver is an inborn, biological need and that a meaningful relationship is first and foremost a physiological process. Each of us is born with a predisposition to become attached to our caregivers, and this biological need becomes a psychological process as each babe develops their sense of self in a specific context. This close early relationship is essential in order to create what is now called a "secure base" in the world, a sense of place and belonging that is as necessary as food and water for human beings to thrive (Bowlby, 1980; 1988).

Right at the end of World War II, British psychoanalysis was in serious conflict, with some, especially the Kleinians, exclusively concerned with the child's internal psychic structures and phantasy life. Internal conflicts were thought to be a result of Freud's universal drive conditions. Others, as I mentioned when I talked about the middle school, were increasingly focused on the outer reality of the child's life and explaining why certain family conditions caused certain children to become disturbed. Freud had abandoned his sexual trauma theory in favor of the child's imagination, but Bowlby asserted that emotional contact and continuity of care were both key to psychological health. Few listened at the time.

In the 1940s, Bowlby and his collaborators had two organically occurring groups of children to study. Because of the Blitz (1940–1941), children had been evacuated from London and transported to safer areas for the duration of the war. Without exception, they all hated it—children and parents alike. That was his first group. As noted earlier in discussing René Spitz, at that time, hospitals forbade parents from staying with their sick children. The nursing staff noted that each time parents left, the children became upset—we now would say that they protested—and they concluded that it would be easier to keep the parents away so that the children would be less upset, creating his second living example of what happens when children and parents are inappropriately separated.

In these live situations, Bowlby and his students discovered a predictable pattern of first "protest," then "despair" (collapse), and finally, if the separation were too long, "detachment." He realized that for a young child separation anxiety is unbearable, wordless, and the foundation for all future anxieties. It was the counterpoint to the infant's need for positive fusion created by continuity of care. For Bowlby, separation anxiety is the root of most psychological disturbance. He further noted that all of these painful states are accompanied by measurable bodily changes, such as a lower, more erratic heart rate (Bowlby, 1969; Karen, 1994). Later, researchers documented several important physiological measures of too much separation, including cortisol regulation and hippocampal development (Gerhardt, 2004).

Once the child falls into detachment, he can appear socially normal again and will accept other caregivers, which is what generally happened in the hospital. Since the need to survive is paramount, creating a false self of looking and acting normal is the path to survival. After a prolonged separation, when the young child is returned to his parents or other primary caregivers, he typically will not accept them; sometimes he will not even recognize them. What follows is a process of alternate clinging and detachment. With persistence on the part of the parents, he might well accept and eventually re-attach to them, or he might never feel that deep safety and sense of being real ever again.

Bowlby noted that partial deprivation of continuous care could result in either excessive need for love or for revenge, while complete deprivation resulted in listlessness, quiet unresponsiveness, and retardation of development. Assuming the child survived, this condition resulted in superficiality of expression, lack of real feeling, failure in concentration, and inclination towards deceit and compulsive behaviors (Bowlby, 1969).

Delinquent behavior

Ironically, both Bowlby and Winnicott published papers in the 1940s proposing that juvenile delinquents had suffered serious interpersonal losses prior to exhibiting their troubling behavior and that these deficits might be a cause of those delinquent behaviors. True to his approach, Bowlby conducted a study comparing juvenile thieves in a clinic environment with a control group and found that the group that had broken the law had suffered significantly more maternal deprivation. For him, the objective facts speak for themselves and society must listen and change (Bowlby, 1944). True to his experience as both an analyst and pediatrician, Winnicott was interested in the inner meaning created by outer experience. He wrote about the need for all children to be antisocial in their search for boundaries and that if they don't find boundaries in the family they will search further afield into the society at large. When the family does not provide properly for the child, the child will turn to antisocial behaviors as a substitute for parental care (Winnicott, 1946). For Winnicott, this is a form of hope. Winnicott was always interested in the subjective processes and the unconscious meanings and consequences of external events, while Bowlby focused on the external lived experience of his patients. Today, we acknowledge both lenses are true and necessary. Trauma is real and how it is internalized creates the suffering we are trying to relieve.

Secure attachment to a secure base

With a responsive caregiver, an infant develops what is now called "secure attachment," including a "secure base," which is created through timely and affectionate care. This secure base—an external, usually adult caregiver—offers bodily connection in a reliable, safe fashion that soothes and vitalizes the infant (Bowlby, 1988). Additionally, the secure base offers a mind that holds the baby internally and communicates through actions: "I have a mind, and you have a mind, and together we can manage any upset you may be having" (Fonagy, 2001).

Protest

Once this secure base is established, the baby can explore, play, and most easily learn, developing mental and motor skills rapidly. In this context, the baby can create, imagine, relax, and enjoy. Of equal importance, with secure attachment, they also can protest in an effort to get their real needs met. This aspect of secure attachment is less pleasurable for the parents, but it is critically important. If protest is disallowed, the baby is forced into either chronic anger or submission (the root of Winnicott's compliance or Brandchaft's pathological accommodation). Additionally, the individuation journey is waylaid because the child is forced to react to an external demand either by conforming or rebelling, rather than responding to her own inner callings (Gerhardt, 2004).

When Jess and I sit quietly together, we are waiting for her words, needs, and thoughts to emerge. It is clear from her personal style that Jess did not protest when it would have been appropriate. She has never rebelled in any way. She has always conformed to the needs of others. In the beginning of our work, it was unthinkable for her to speak out in her family, but now it is actually doable. She notes with pride and healthy self-esteem that she can insist that her large extended family wait for her to find her words. She can even insist sometimes that things be done her way. She is beginning to feel equally entitled to make some of the big decisions in her family, not just to execute the wishes of others. In finding her protest, she has reignited her growth process and her excitement in life.

Working model

Bowlby developed what he called the "internal working model," which includes expectations about both the self and the other. Among these expectations are: Am I lovable? Will others welcome me and be interested in me? Will others care for me and even take care of me? Will others help me? (Bowlby, 1988)

The baby's caregiver carries their own internal working model of how their world works. Nonverbally and non-consciously, they share their model of intimacy and expectations with the baby. Slowly, the baby will create their own internal working model, which will be an amalgam of their experiences with all of their important others.

Bowlby called these "working" or "representational" models because he knew they would change over time. He realized that inner life is an ongoing process. Babies form their first set of expectations of how the world works from their primary caregivers. The more secure attachment the more flexible the inner working model and more able to change and meet new circumstances. When the mother is consistently less available or attuned, these working models become fixed and also inappropriate to current life situations (Bowlby, 1988). Over time, their own expectations of how valuable or worthy of care they are will influence the others around them, creating all the dances of intimacy—both healthy and unhealthy—that form their relational life. Of course, it is very important for each therapist to know his own personal working model, which will be part of the dance between him and his patients.

By around two years of age, the baby has a rudimentary knowledge of "theory of mind," that innate ability to know the inner states of others, including their intentions (Fonagy et al., 2004). We all read the face and body language of others to discern their basic feelings. In this sense, both mother and baby read the mind of the other. Through lived experience, each knows that the other has beliefs and desires that may be contradictory to their own beliefs and desires. Furthermore, both know when others are "pretending" and then can enter into created imaginary worlds for play, exploration, and escape.

Loss and abandonment anxiety

Within attachment theory, loss of connection from the critically important caring other is central to human emotional distress. Abandonment anxiety is considered a major root of all of the mood disorders and, if severe enough, the root of the more vulnerable character disorders (Bowlby, 1988; Karen, 1994; Gerhardt, 2004). To be fully abandoned as a tiny baby would be to die. As adults, all forms of rejection and loss can trigger our basic need for reassurance that we are connected to important others. If there is too much loss at too young an age, the child will feel victimized by implicit, nonverbal, and unconscious feelings that cannot be processed or managed. Even in healthy adults, overwhelming feelings require an external other for processing and integration. Such loss creates a host of psychological issues, including depression, anxiety, panic attacks, and the psychosomatic expressions of psychic pain. Currently, in alignment with Bromberg, the relational school, and the intersubjective school, the attachment school would agree with the neuroscience term "activation" or "dysregulated" (Schore, 2012). If too much happens too young, grief becomes unbearable and stays stuck in some bodily or non-conscious form. The capacity to mourn and to integrate loss and grief is considered to be a developmental achievement critical to adult functioning. A young child lacks the words and skills to integrate such terrible feelings, which is why an external regulating presence is so crucial in childhood. Furthermore, Bowlby suggests that if there has been traumatic separation with too many substitutes—that is, insufficient specific caring—the child could well be unable to develop meaningful relationships in later life (Bretherton, 1995). Mourning these lost early attachments is an important aspect of therapy and each therapist must develop his own capacity to welcome and not push away the intense emotional suffering of these losses.

> *When he is stressed, my client Jack "falls apart." In modern language, he is easily dysregulated. Jack struggles to create safety for himself, both interpersonally and intra-psychically. When he needs to travel for work, he becomes terribly anxious, even phobic, that something terrible will happen if he leaves the safety of his home. Jack does not connect this fear of leaving home with abandonment anxiety. Instead, he protects himself with a layer of anger—at himself; at his job for its demands; and at me because, so far, the fear has not lessened. I believe that the anger protects him from the grief and mourning. His more superficial yet very intense fury protects him from falling into a hole from which he believes he might never emerge. Only as we co-create some trust in our relationship is Jack able to peek below his anger into other, deeper feelings, including his fear he might lose me due to his intense emotional reactions.*

Starting with Bowlby, current attachment literature has much to say about the optimal conditions for children—theory of mind, the importance of healthy protest, and the devastating effect of loss as central to human distress. These issues have been studied across cultures and are now considered to be universal. Attachment theory research has created a model that includes secure attachment (mentioned above) and two varieties of insecure attachment, which represent solutions to non-optimal care. An "ambivalent attachment" style is characterized by over-dependence on important others. An individual with an "avoidant attachment" style denies his needs and refuses to openly connect with a needed other. These remind me very much of Balint's two unconscious solutions (Chapter 5) to discovering that merger and oneness are illusions. In addition to the two insecure styles, there is an extreme category referred to as "disorganized/dysregulated attachment," which is highly dysfunctional. We can think of human pathology as falling into these categories (Bowlby, 1988; Karen, 1994). We now assume that the need to attach is a universal biological given. Each style tends to carry forward in time, affecting the quality of adult relationships and, therefore, the quality of life each individual achieves.

Bowlby was very clear about how to conduct a therapy. For him, the therapist is a companion, not an authority with interpretations. He notes that it is the job of the patient to find his own way into his inner life, including understanding his family dynamics. He is very much an optimist, believing that the human psyche tends toward growth and healing given the best environment possible (Bowlby, 1988). This is more a part of the humanistic tradition than the classical one.

MARY AINSWORTH

Among the most important of the Bowlby collaborators was Mary Ainsworth (1913–1999). Born and educated in Canada, she later studied with Bowlby in London. Ainsworth had a mind that loved organization and understood the importance of the scientific method, including statistical analysis. She was not content with generalizing from a few cases and changed the landscape of developmental research with her rigor (Ainsworth et al., 1978). During the 1950s, she went to Uganda to research attachment and weaning patterns in an extensive longitudinal study. At this time, determining attachment style required an observer to conduct multiple interviews with both child and parents. Thus, these first forays into understanding attachment, whether in England or Africa, were very time-consuming and required extensive resources. In order to pursue her research, Ainsworth overcame multiple difficulties, both personal and professional, including learning the local language. Eventually, she published what remains an important classic in both ethnology and child development. Ainsworth (1967) observed the same patterns in the Ugandan village as she did in England, thereby consolidating the idea that the need for attachment is universal and that children will attach to whoever cares for them, no matter how well or how poorly.

By 1965, Ainsworth had returned to North America, where she designed the "strange situation," outlined below. This model shifted the study of attachment from conducting fieldwork in homes and villages to spending less than an hour in a controlled laboratory situation (Karen, 1994). The study of attachment, in all of its forms, flourished as a result. Due to the ongoing efforts of Ainsworth and many others, attachment theory became a solid research model for understanding child development as a contextual process (Ainsworth et al., 1978; Bretherton, 1995).

Strange situation and categories of attachment

Currently, researchers outline four types of attachment, and all are measured using the laboratory technique called the strange situation (Ainsworth et al., 1978). Traditionally, in the experiment the child and mother enter a playroom and begin to play with the toys. Then, a stranger enters the playroom and, after a while (time is dependent on the age of the child), the mother leaves, and the observers watch the child's reactions to being left. The observers are very interested in how the child handles the mother's leaving—that is, separation—and how he handles her return. Can he reunite, indicating trust in their ongoing relationship and, therefore, secure attachment? If not, the nature of the child's reaction will determine which of the insecure categories apply to him (Ainsworth et al., 1978; Karen, 1994).

If the child falls into the secure category, he protests the mom's leaving, making it clear she is needed and special. However, after a few minutes, he returns to playing, perhaps relating to the stranger if he offers to play or interact with the child. When mom returns, the child is delighted to see her and, after a brief reunion, returns to playing. This is the best early beginning, allowing the child a sense of trust that they can manage upset and that the world is relatively trustworthy and ongoing.

If the child falls into the ambivalent category, his protest over mom's leaving is, generally, much more impassioned. The stranger finds it hard to soothe the child and get him back to playing. When mom returns, she also cannot soothe him. The child alternates between clinging to her and pushing her away, perhaps even hitting her. The two cannot get settled. Ambivalent attachment style appears to be related to a generally unreliable and/or under-involved approach to caregiving.

If the child falls into the avoidant category, he does not protest the mom's leaving and appears unconcerned over her absence. Perhaps he notes it and then continues playing on his own. He appears independent of needing her. When she returns, he acts as if she doesn't matter to him. Avoidant attachment is correlated with intrusive, excessively stimulating, and controlling interactions with a caregiver or by a caregiver who demands that the child prematurely be an adult.

The fourth category became apparent later in their research. Some infants experienced fear while looking at their mother's face or even being around her mood. Eventually, these infants were said to have disorganized or disorienting or dysregulated attachment. More will be said of this in the next section on Mary Main.

Ainsworth, Main, and countless others have done innumerable studies using the strange situation at various ages comparing securely attached children with all of the insecure types, hoping to both find predictive measures of mental health and viable interventions (Ainsworth et al, 1978; Main, 2000). I would say, at this point, the research is suggestive but inconclusive. Sometimes there is a high correlation between the style of the 9-month-old, the 6-year-old, and the 18-year-old. But a lot of life has intervened, including the father and other relatives, maybe a good teacher, and of course adolescence. Some of these have contributed to well-being, others have been disorganizing. Main (2000) does note in her longitudinal research that the secure dyads speak more easily and fluidly with each other and invite real, wide-ranging conversations throughout life. This alone suggests to me that they have more positive connections in later life and, therefore, a higher quality of life.

Additional observations

Extensive research has demonstrated that cortisol levels are higher in children who display insecure attachment patterns when in the strange situation. Additionally, animal studies indicate that repeated hyperarousal actually destroys brain tissue (Gerhardt, 2004). With disorganized attachment, the child develops multiple, segregated, incompatible working models of attachment. Dissociative processes are at work, which is the hallmark of all types of trauma. Furthermore, disorganized attachment may be antecedent to both personality disorders and dissociative identity disorder, which is one of the most serious character disturbances (Fonagy, 2004; Bromberg, 2011).

MARY MAIN

Mary Main, a contemporary American and a student of Ainsworth, has made many contributions to the attachment theory literature, most particularly on adults and the least-secure attachment style. Like Ainsworth, she is a research scientist, wanting theory to be corroborated by statistics and studies. The two extensions that are most valuable to me clinically are her addition of the disorganized/disorienting attachment style (mentioned above) and her Adult Attachment Interview.

All of the researchers had a few children in their studies that were "unclassifiable": children who did not develop an organized defensive pattern to deal with the stresses of separation. The avoidant child shifts his attention away from the potential threat, and the ambivalent child becomes preoccupied, even clingy. Main (1995) went looking for the characteristics of this small, unclassified sample by reviewing notes and videotapes from several studies. She found that some children never develop a cohesive strategy for dealing with distress. Main noticed that, for some of her young research subjects, the mother was actually frightening.

In this situation, the baby is in a terrible dilemma. The person they are supposed to go to for safety and comfort is a person who is consistently unreliable and, in some cases, terrifying. Main and Ainsworth agreed that there was a need for a fourth category, which they designated as disorganized/disorienting. In these instances, the child displays contradictory behavior patterns sequentially or simultaneously. His movements are undirected, incomplete, or interrupted; he falls into repetitive patterns, perhaps freezing or exhibiting apprehension. The child needs care, but this caregiver is frightening; therefore, there is no solution. Biologically, they are compelled to approach the caregiver for care, but this child has learned that approaching the caregiver is unlikely to be satisfying and possibly dangerous (Main, 1995; Gerhardt, 2004). Thus, the terrible dilemma. Subjectively, this last category might be represented by one of my client's poignant words: "My mother? I never occurred to her. I can react to her as an adult, but never dare initiate—you just don't know what you are going to get."

Adult Attachment Inventory

In the 1980s, Main turned her attention to the parents of the children she was studying and created the Adult Attachment Interview (AAI) (Main, 2000; Siegel & Hartzell, 2003). She was and still is interested in longitudinal research to enable both clinicians and public policymakers to help children on all levels. Initially, she used this instrument to document the attachment style the parent had with his own parents, the baby's grandparents. Participating parents are asked in several different ways to describe their own attachment experiences and to evaluate aspects of their current life, including how they parent (Main, 2000).

The AAI is a powerful and effective instrument for understanding adult attachment styles (Siegel & Hartzell, 2003; Siegel, 2008). A skilled practitioner conducts a structured interview, which, among other questions, asks the participant to offer five adjectives to describe his relationship with each of his parents as well as personal stories to back up those adjectives. For all of the insecure attachment styles, this is a very difficult task. Main's research demonstrates that the more secure the attachment, the easier it is for individuals to share their inner world in a logical and coherent fashion, suggesting trust and security. Secure attachment also is highly correlated with the capacity to speak directly and be self-reflective. It is associated with neither compliance nor competitiveness. It correlates positively with high self-esteem, the capacity to value the care provided by others, and to act autonomously.

Main calls the ambivalent style of childhood "preoccupied" in adulthood, and the avoidant style "dismissive" (Main, 1995; Karen, 1994; Siegel & Hartzell, 2003). In my experience, these words accurately describe adults with insecure attachment styles and how they manage their needs for connection and relationship. The individual with a preoccupied style needs a lot of reassurance and closeness. During psychotherapy sessions, these clients thrive with mirroring, conveying that they are valued and understood. In their romantic relationships, they need ongoing physical and sexual contact, both for pleasure and excitement and for the reassurance that they are valued and, most critically, will not be abandoned. They frequently have a tipping point, where they feel invaded and controlled. At that moment, they will push the other away energetically and/or verbally. An individual with a dismissive style needs distance and freedom within their relationships. They demonstrate less emotional connection to their therapists but can be very committed to the work. In their love relationships, they often enjoy parallel living or time apart, needing space and freedom to feel safe and good. They tend to dismiss any strong need of other people, considering it dependency and weakness.

Main's research continues the premise put forth by Ainsworth: A parent's attachment style is highly correlated with the attachment style of their children, at least at the binary level of secure–insecure. Securely attached individuals create securely attached children, and insecurely attached parents create less securely attached children.

Of course, real people don't fall neatly into four boxes, but the four attachment styles are a very useful initial roadmap for understanding the connections a person is willing and able to create. It also suggests how to best approach different clients. What is reassuring for an ambivalent style might be impinging for an avoidant style.

Dan is a good example of an avoidant attachment style. He has a few friends that he sees irregularly, and they are almost never mentioned during our time together. When he returns from a visit to his parents, he has little to report regarding his interactions with them. He says he loves them and that they are good people. Yet there are no intimate conversations, no problem-solving discussions. He can talk sports with his dad and tell his mom about his writing projects, but he is slightly relieved to be headed home on Sunday evening.

Earned secure

Main's research generated a new category of attachment style, called "earned secure." In some cases, when the child's attachment style created in a given family was less than secure, positive experiences with others, such as neighbors, teachers, mentors, and psychotherapists, can create the trust necessary for a more secure sense of self to emerge in the adult, with its characteristic relaxation and creativity and enhanced trust in others. Of course, this is one way of looking at the goals of good psychotherapy or any individuation path. Trust, connection, and security are necessary for individual well-being, and all three of the insecure patterns inhibit these possibilities. The pain of loneliness and crippling psychopathology are highly correlated with insecure attachment styles (Roisman et al., 2002; Siegel & Hartzell, 2003).

Today, all but the most classical forms of psychoanalysis recognize the importance of attachment, even as they attend to it differently within their own theoretical stances. The Bowlby lineage, along with the work on early childhood development of Daniel Stern and Beatrice Beebe, has had an immeasurable impact on both theory and practice of psychoanalysis and psychotherapy in general. Most psychotherapists and anyone who works with children would agree with the idea captured by Thomas Lewis: "Stability means finding people who regulate you well and staying near them" (Lewis et al., 2000).

PETER FONAGY

Peter Fonagy is currently the most acclaimed clinician-scholar integrating psychoanalysis and attachment theory. A native of Hungary, he is head of the Anna Freud National Centre for Children and Families, based in London. He writes that secure attachment is the bedrock of human development, enabling a sense of both self and other to develop. He maintains that secure attachment precedes the capacities outlined by the psychoanalytic traditions, such as reality testing, symbolization, and moral development (Fonagy et al., 2004).

In addition to linking these two traditions, Fonagy insists that all psychotherapy must ground itself through solid research. Does a particular form of treatment work? How can we measure results? His specialized areas of research are borderline personality disorder, early attachment relationships, and violence.

Mentalization

From his clinical work and research, Fonagy and his collaborators have put forth the concept of "mentalization." It is through secure attachment that each of us learns to mentalize and regulate our feelings and physiology. This means we can make and use mental representations of our own and other people's emotional states. The various insecure attachment styles leave children unable to manage

(continued)

(continued)

themselves, particularly under stressful situations, and often unable to "read" and be empathic to others. The consequences of these deficits are dire, leading to isolation and loneliness as well as serious psychopathology in severe cases. Fonagy's solution is called mentalization-based treatment or therapy: Patients receive appropriate mirroring for their emotional life as well as clear guidance on creating real relationships with real others, either in a hospital setting or the consulting room (Fonagy et al., 2004).

Fonagy has published many studies and books comparing various parenting styles, resultant attachment issues, and healing prototypes. Clearly, he belongs to the attachment tradition while being solidly steeped in classical psychoanalysis: The better the early attachment, the better a person is able to envision the mental states of others as well as himself. Moreover, the self exists only in the context of others, and the development of a self in childhood is an accumulation of the child's experiences of self-in-relationship. These lived experiences are then abstracted into internal representations or internal working models. In his understanding, the core issue is the caregiver's ability to communicate to the child that she understands and cares about his unique needs, emotions, and intentions. This transmission is a nonverbal but clearly understandable process, whereby the child signals and the mother interprets, usually adding language to the communication. This consequent "theory of mind" is a key determinant of self-organization and, later, well-being (Fonagy et al., 2004).

Attachment style and theory of mind

Among Fonagy's many research findings is that a mother's attachment classification before the birth of her child is an excellent predictor of that mother–child attachment pattern (Fonagy et al., 1991). Anything predictive is very exciting to both the clinical community and the public health community. The parent's overall sensitivity to her child—her capacity to envision her child as a separate, sentient being even before its birth—predicts both the child's attachment style and his mentalization capacity. Winnicott knew this to be true and wrote of it in a different language. Fonagy and his team have published many studies outlining precisely how the sensitive mother thinks about her baby. Her thinking shapes her behavior, and the babe internalizes her behavior as their sense of self. The baby of a sensitive mother concludes, "I am valuable, and my needs are understandable." These are the wholesome messages conveyed by her behaviors (Winnicott's holding and handling) when she is with him. When she is not in his presence, she continues to hold him in her thoughts and in her imagination. Over time, the babe begins to be able to hold her in his imagination; thus, in secure attachment, the child can let the mother out of sight without undue distress. He has learned to hold her and remember her from inside (Fonagy et al., 2004).

Fonagy (2004) further notes a correlation between secure attachment and slightly imperfect attunement. This supports Kohut's notion of curative cycles of disruption and repair (as beautifully researched by Beebe). Here, small, manageable failures in attunement that are quickly repaired actually create the possibility of reliability, trust, and more secure attachment. Fonagy's research concludes that both affect tracking and marking with small degrees of difference can promote growth, so long as they occur in the ongoing context of mutual attunement and regulation. We might well call this context care or even love.

Marking

Another of Fonagy's contributions is the idea of "marking." Here, the caregiver attunes herself to and actively imitates the infant's affect through facial, vocal, and postural expression. But the caregiver "marks" her mirroring by a slight exaggeration, thus providing the infant with an experience of attunement along with a hint that the mirroring comes from an outside other. By both matching the infant's affective expression and, at the same time, marking herself as different, the caregiver manages to present both regulatory attunement—I see you—and recognized difference and separateness—I am not you—within a single interaction (Fonagy et al, 2004).

Interpersonal neurobiology

In order to bring psychoanalysis into the modern world, we must have some understanding of the new discipline, interpersonal neurobiology. I will discuss the three who have presented at psychoanalytic conferences and written the most, influencing all forms of psychotherapy by offering research and language to ground invisible feelings in interpersonal, neurological interactions.

ALLAN SCHORE

One of the most important contributors to the modern scene, American psychiatrist and researcher Allan Schore is a leader in the new disciplines of neuropsychology and interpersonal neurobiology. He regularly presents his work on affect regulation at psychoanalytic and trauma conferences, seeking to move all forms of psychotherapy towards a more scientific stance. Schore studies brain research at a biological level, and he also is devoted to attachment theory, along with all the data it integrates.

Brain development

In our current understanding, our modern human brain developed in stages, over the eons. We share our hindbrain with most other animals; it is the part of the brain that manages our physiology, our perceptions, our physical being. It also controls our most primitive defenses: an automatic scanning for danger and freeze/faint responses to threats we perceive as life threatening. We share our limbic brain—small structures in the middle of our brain—with all mammals. It controls our attachment needs, our need for play, and our capacity to decide between fight or flight. In comparison to other mammals, our neocortex, or new brain, is huge. This is the source of our capacity for abstract thinking, future planning, and moral development. Critically, unlike the hindbrain and midbrain, the neocortex is not fully formed at birth. How it will form is dependent on interactions with the human environment.

This neocortex is divided into a right and left hemisphere. These have different functions, and each perceives the world differently. According to both Schore and Siegel, the right matures ahead of the left and is the source of emotional processing and holistic images of both inner and outer reality. The left hemisphere controls language and linear, logical thinking. It is usually dominant in adults (Schore, 2012; Siegel, 2008).

Schore (2012) has written extensively on the uneven development of the right and left hemispheres of the brain. He notes that the right hemisphere develops ahead of the left, and it is responsible for emotional processes and seeing the whole interpersonal picture in a "bodily felt sense." For Schore, the right brain is the biological substrate of Freud's unconscious, and he emphasizes the power of that unconscious just as Freud did but in very different ways. Because the right hemisphere develops ahead of the left, Schore concludes that emotions are more foundational to our sense of self and well-being than the words and logic of the left brain. His research and reasoning conclude that our sense of self, and all of our implicit processing of the interpersonal world, are processed in the early-maturing right brain. His research substantiates that the development of the neocortex is experience-dependent; it unfolds within a context that quite literally shapes it (Schore, 2012; Gerhardt, 2004). Of course, genetic factors still matter, but Schore maintains that the nature–nurture controversy is a false dichotomy, as genes and environment are interrelating from the moment of conception.

In Schore's therapeutic model (2012), attuned communication is right brain to right brain. That is, at a nonverbal and unconscious level, we are all scanning our human environments, especially the human face, to find safety and connection (Porges, 2004). Ekman (2003) has proven that we read faces non-consciously in milliseconds and act on this information non-consciously all the time. From this viewpoint, psychotherapy is much more about connection and creating safety than it is about words and interpretations. For Schore, an individual's capacity to regulate their bodily feelings and affects begins during babyhood in interaction with an attuned caregiver. Over time, a child incorporates the wider world so that groups and even culture act at the unconscious psychobiological level in a continuous flow.

Schore's detailed and scholarly works outline the world of affect regulation, beginning with the impact of the surrounding world on the very young child and continuing into adult development. He elucidates how early attachment trauma affects the right hemisphere and the limbic system throughout life. He demonstrates this theory with neuro-imaging, showing the physical and observable effects of such interactions within the brain. For him, all forms of psychopathology are forms of affect dysregulation, and all forms of psychotherapy are forms of affect regulation. He further maintains that eliminating negative states is not sufficient for well-being. Just as the "good enough mother"—the mother who creates secure attachment—amplifies positive states in her baby, enlivens him, and encourages his excitement and curiosity, good therapy should also enhance and champion the positive side of life (Schore, 2012). By the beginning of the 21st century, researchers and practitioners alike are clear that human well-being involves finding the people who regulate you well and keeping them near.

DANIEL SIEGEL

My next choice in this lineage is American psychiatrist and researcher Daniel Siegel. In a prolific series of books and articles written over the last two decades, he has put forth an elegant theory of human development and psychotherapy. His audiobook, *The Neurobiology of "We"*, is perhaps the clearest distillation of his clinical theory and practice rooted in neurobiology, attachment theory, and mindfulness from the spiritual traditions of meditation. He also writes revealingly about himself as a person, parent, and psychiatrist. He brings both scholarship and great compassion to his writings and to his patients. Siegel, like Schore, brings us firmly into the world of modern neuroscience, where the brain-mind can be studied both objectively and subjectively. Both Schore and Siegel maintain that the brain is neuroplastic, that is, able to change and grow throughout life (Schore, 2012; Siegel, 2010).

Modern mindfulness

Modern mindfulness is a translation of a spiritual practice first created eons ago by Eastern mystics in order to achieve enlightenment or "at oneness with all." By deeply focusing on first the breath and then the thoughts and feelings that arise as one sits quietly, a practitioner can calm himself into various transcendent states. In its modern iteration, attending to the breath is used to calm the emotional states of stress and negative feelings. Siegel offers several versions of mindfulness practices, paying attention first to the breath and then to thoughts around the self and significant others. Practicing mindfulness is positively correlated with healthy brain development, stress alleviation, well-being, and the development of compassion (Siegel, 2010).

Like Stern before him, Siegel is very interested in the idea of "emergent." In the 1980s, Stern wrote that the infant has an emergent sense of self (Stern, 1985). Siegel believes that the mind itself is an emergent property located between two separate others. For him, the mind is no longer only located in a skull; rather, it is an ongoing co-creation between two others. In his definition, the mind is the flow of energy and information within a person and between two people (Siegel, 2008; 2010). Furthermore, the mind is capable of being studied subjectively by paying attention, slowing down, and looking inward. This is his form of mindfulness. He talks about it as making friends with yourself and with your mind.

Siegel also is a rigorous scientist, and he uses experiments and imaging equipment to research his ideas. He in no way denies that psychotherapy is an art—even a spiritual art—but he suggests that there are better and worse ways of conducting a therapy to help those who are suffering. He believes in compassion and kindness. His theory proposes that our big brains evolved in order to read the minds of others, so as to be able to cooperate in large, non-biologically-related groups. The part of the brain that reads others is called the middle prefrontal cortex. This also is the same part of the brain that develops in mindfulness meditation, as shown by functional MRI studies studying long-term meditators at the University of Wisconsin (Goleman & Davidson, 2017). Siegel notes parallels among secure attachment, mindful awareness, and the relationship between therapist and patient. With colleagues, he has conducted a number of studies exploring the relationship of secure attachment between parent and child and the effective therapeutic relationship between clinician and patient. He maintains that each promotes the growth of fibers in the prefrontal part of the brain. He also teaches both his students and his patients mindfulness in order to develop the integrative powers of the prefrontal cortex (Siegel & Hartzell, 2003; Siegel, 2010).

Again, like Stern, Siegel's focus is often on attunement. The good enough mother attunes to her child, and the good enough therapist must do the same. When mother is attuned, the child is able to feel good about himself, manage his needs, and connect with others when he wants to. When secure attachment is missing, it is the

Middle prefrontal cortex

Siegel's study of the middle prefrontal cortex has led him to the following set of considerations: The functions of this part of the brain are to regulate your body, balance your emotions, attune to others, modulate fear, respond to situations flexibly, and to practice empathy. These completely overlap with the positive findings of secure attachment. Two other human skills are very important in the mindfulness literature but have only recently been studied in the attachment literature. These are intuition and morality. According to Siegel, these also overlap with attachment research findings (Siegel, 2010).

work of the therapy to jump-start the natural processes thwarted by the anxieties of insecure attachment.

Following these thinkers and their research, I now see therapy as a reflective dialogue, focusing mutual attention on one side of the equation—the patient—while paying mindful attention to the therapist's inner life. Through mindfulness, the attachment literature, and modern neuroscience, Siegel has come to the same conclusions that the later self psychologists and the relational school did. Therapy and psychoanalysis are a two-person event, both therapist and patient must participate fully in the present moment, each bringing their personal sense of self to the meeting. Siegel, like Schore, is clear that the emotional part of us—the right brain and the limbic system—is the main driver of change and growth; the narrative of the linear logical left brain is key for communicating one mind to another. As an ideal, this is the "I–thou" of Martin Buber. Both will be affected and both will be changed by the encounter.

All of this information and these ideas affect how I practice psychotherapy. As I noted at the very beginning of this book, the way a person enters my office is always significant. I can focus on my innate, unconscious capacity to read the face and the body language of each person. Once I have consciously used myself to read the face and the body, I can make an educated guess about the mood, even the emotions. At the same time, I need to read myself, not only for my feelings and preoccupations but also for my specific feelings about this client at this appointment. Am I welcoming? If not, why? Am I slightly irritated about something that happened between us last time? Is this an encounter I am actually not looking forward to? Did I get irritated last time and show that irritation either appropriately or inappropriately? These are the swirls within each of us that are coming together with the conscious intent of understanding something going on in the client, as well as transforming or healing some part of suffering. Of course, all of the unconscious needs and desires are still to be discovered by each of us and within each of us.

I often don't look forward to my time with Dan, as his frozen qualities have been difficult for me to melt and find ways to deeply engage him. For me, my therapeutic task is to welcome him into my psychic space. It is easy for me to be curious about him, but it is more difficult to find ways of engaging him, creating a sustaining connection that we both value. In the language of neuroscience, I am clear that my intention and my left brain are welcoming, the question is the felt sense of the right brain. Does he feel relaxed, safe, welcomed when I know I am a little stiff inside? Can I open myself to be with him more deeply, more emotionally? I do know that he comes regularly and will find a way to reschedule if he can't make our normal time. I read this as a good sign, that he is getting some of what he wants from our time together, even he if cannot speak more fluently about his inner life or our relationship yet.

STEPHEN PORGES

Stephen Porges is another neuroscientist presenting at clinical conferences, specifically those focused on trauma. His laboratory research has revealed that our vagal nerve has three very different branches serving very different psychological safety mechanisms (Porges, 2017; Porges & Dana, 2018). He proposes that at our highest functioning, using our most evolved vagal nerve, we enable a complex relational style called "social engagement," involving face reading, the tilt of our head, the gestures of our hands, the regulation of our heart. Under threat, we move to the biological givens of "fight or flight," using another branch of that same nerve: We get angry, we argue, we bargain, we pretend, we deny. We are threatened; we are looking for safety and even hoping to re-create a safe relationship. Under a third dramatic and traumatic circumstance, we call upon our neurological ability to freeze or faint using the most primitive branch of the same nerve: This is our inbuilt capacity to psychologically dissociate, to emotionally "leave" a situation that is overwhelming or unbearable while staying physically present (Geller & Porges, 2014; Porges, 2017).

Porges' research has demonstrated that these three options are built into our nervous system through the vagus nerve. Among other things, social engagement involves our preference from birth to gaze at the human face, our capacity to make eye contact, and our wiring to hear the pitch of the human voice. Fight and flight involve an activated sympathetic nervous system allowing fear-driven movement, either bodily or psychologically. The freeze/faint response calls upon our physiological capacity through the parasympathetic system to shut down bodily functions while still staying alive. He is clear that these are among the biological systems that underpin our psychological defenses (Porges, 2015; 2017).

I find all of these layers of neurological functioning helpful when sitting with clients, but I am especially grateful to have a neurological understanding of dissociation. I now understand that dissociation always points to terror and trauma, often relational trauma. The freeze/faint response is totally non-voluntary; once in its grip, in the shutdown controlled by the parasympathetic nervous system, it is very difficult to directly intervene. It is a very slow process, involving tracking feelings as they move through the body in order to find words to express the terror the dissociation is protecting.

"Ruth" struggled with dissociated aspects of herself. She spent her first three years of life alone with her mother. When her father returned from the Vietnam War, he was not happy to have a daughter. Whatever his motivations and/or war trauma, he openly and continuously shamed and verbally abused Ruth. Her mother never protected her. When I met Ruth, she had endured two abusive marriages, and was currently divorced and raising her children as a single parent. She was an extremely nonverbal participant in our work together, usually sitting on the edge of her chair and staring into space. Occasionally, a tremor would go through her. In my experience, she was somewhere else, seeing, hearing,

and sensing other events as if they were happening in the room in the present moment. It took a long time for us to create enough safety to locate the sensations in her body and describe the images that she was experiencing. It took longer still for the words to build a scene from her past. Ruth could disappear into altered states and these dissociated aspects for long moments. She would startle when I asked, "What are you seeing or hearing right now?" Then it would take silence and waiting before she could find words to express memories from her childhood, from her marriages, and from previous therapies. Slowly, Ruth gathered herself, allowing us to share the horror of her past and grieve for her lost childhood and adult suffering.

By following the attachment thread of psychoanalysis, we have reached 21st-century neuroscience and what is currently called interpersonal neurobiology. All of our theories and practices change if we incorporate these ideas. The unconscious is real, is pre-reflective; that is, it is what happens in the first years of life before words and memory are available. Emotions are primary and must first be regulated by caring others. Through that mostly nonverbal dance between baby and caregiver, we each gather a sense of self—a sense of going-on-being in Winnicott language, and self-continuity in Stern language. As our sense of self was created in an interpersonal matrix, so is the domain of healing. Relational trauma creates insecure attachment and only another relationship, an attuned and caring relationship, can modify that attachment style.

Key concepts Chapter 8

Abandonment or separation anxiety – the intense panic experienced when separated from the mother for too long; now considered the source of much psychological suffering in adults

Adult Attachment Inventory – the structured interview devised by Main to determine an adult's attachment style; used extensively by Siegel in his work integrating psychotherapy and mindfulness

Ambivalent attachment style – an insecure style involving both clinging to and rejecting others

Attachment theory – Bowlby's assertion that the infant needs consistent care in order to develop physically and psychologically

Avoidant attachment style – an insecure style involves keeping a large emotional distance from significant others

Despair – profound grief, hopelessness, and helplessness; for a baby if separation from the "care-er" is too long, the infant gives up and retreats into himself with a darkened mood

Detachment – the creation of a defense or "false self" to manage the pain of inappropriate separation; the final step of the separation cycle

Dismissive attachment – avoidant attachment in adults, keeping emotional distance

Disorganized/dysregulated attachment – when the caregiver evokes fear rather than safety the baby lives in a terrified state not able to find safety with others or within himself

Earned secure – Main's observation that some adults transform an insecure style of attachment to a more secure style through positive life experiences

Insecure attachment – the dynamic created when the caretaker can't meet enough of the baby's needs; the baby cannot rest in safety

Internal working model – Bowlby's term for the baby's unconscious understanding of the relationship between himself and his "care-er"

Marking – the facial gestures a caregiver makes to help her baby distinguish between his emotional state and hers, as first noted by Fonagy

Mentalization-based treatment – Fonagy's therapy to help people who suffer from disorganized attachment issues to regulate their feelings and thoughts

Mindfulness – a spiritual practice that has been modified to incorporate it into psychotherapy to manage anxiety, reduce stress, and heighten awareness—a core technique in Siegel's work

Preoccupied attachment – ambivalent attachment in adults

Protest – an essential part of the cycle of attachment and separation

Right brain to right brain – Schore's understanding that emotional connection and communication happen through the right side of the brain, nonverbally and unconsciously in both babies and adults. It is the location of effective psychotherapy

Secure attachment – knowing that the "care-er" is reliable and dependable creating inner safety

Secure base – attachment theory's understanding that the external caregiver creates safety and the capacity to thrive in an infant; over time that safety is internalized into an inner secure base

Separation anxiety – the fundamental source of all anxiety—away from the secure base and safety

Social engagement system – Porges' designation of the human preference to gaze at another face, make eye contact, hear the human voice, and gesture to communicate

Strange situation – the laboratory experiment devised by Ainsworth to determine attachment style

Theory of mind – the innate ability to know I have thoughts and feelings and you have thoughts and feelings and when around you I have some idea of your state of being. Was first a philosophical stance and is now a concept researched by developmental psychology

References

Ainsworth, M.D.S. (1967) *Infancy in Uganda: Infant Care and the Growth of Love*. Baltimore, MD: Johns Hopkins University Press.

Ainsworth, M., Blehar, M.C., Waters, E. & Wall, S. (eds). (1978) *Patterns of Attachment*. Hillsdale, NJ: Lawrence Erlbaum.

Bowlby, J. (1944) Forty four juvenile thieves: Their characters and home lives. *International Journal of Psycho-Analysis*, 25: 19–52.

Bowlby, J. (1951) *Maternal Care and Mental Health*. World Health Organization Monograph (Serial No. 2).

Bowlby, J. (1969) *Attachment*. London: Pelican.

Bowlby, J. (1980) *Attachment and Loss*, vol 3: *Loss: Sadness and Depression*. London: Hogarth Press.

Bowlby, J. (1988) *A Secure Base*. New York: Basic Books.

Bretherton, I. (1995) The origins of attachment theory: John Bowlby and Mary Ainsworth. In Goldberg, S., Muir, R., & Kerr, J. (eds) *Attachment Theory: Social, Developmental, and Clinical Perspectives*. Hillsdale, NJ: Analytic Press.

Bromberg, P.M. (2011) *The Shadow of the Tsunami*. New York: Routledge.

Ekman, P. (2003) *Emotions Revealed*. New York: Henry Holt.

Fonagy, P. (2001) *Attachment Theory and Psychoanalysis*. New York: Other Press.

Fonagy, P., Steele, H., & Steele, M. (1991). Maternal representations of attachment during pregnancy predict the organization of infant–mother attachment at one year of age. *Child Development*, 62: 891–905.

Fonagy, P., Gergely, G., Jurist, E., & Target, M. (2004) *Affect Regulation, Mentalization and the Development of the Self*. New York: Other Press.

Geller, S.M. & Porges, S.W. (2014) Therapeutic presence: Neurophysiological mechanisms mediating feeling safe in therapeutic relationships. *Journal of Psychotherapy Integration*, 24 (3): 178–192.

Gerhardt, S. (2004) *Why Love Matters*. New York: Brunner-Routledge.

Goleman, D. & Davidson, R.J. (2017) *Altered Traits: Science Reveals How Meditation Changes Your Mind, Brain, and Body*. New York: Avery, Random House.

Holmes, J. (1995) "Something there is that doesn't love a wall": John Bowlby, attachment theory and psychoanalysis. In Goldberg, S., Muir, R., & Kerr, J. (eds) *Attachment Theory: Social, Developmental, and Clinical Perspectives*. Hillsdale, NJ: Analytic Press.

Karen, R. (1994) *Becoming Attached*. New York: Warner.

Lewis, T., Amini, F., & Lannon, R. (2000) *A General Theory of Love*. New York: Random House.

Main, M. (1995) Recent studies in attachment: Overview, with selected implications for clinical work. In Goldberg, S., Muir, R., & Kerr, J. (ed) *Attachment Theory: Social, Developmental, and Clinical Perspectives*. Hillsdale, NJ: Analytic Press.

Main, M. (2000) The Adult Attachment Interview: Fear, attention, safety and discourse process. *Journal of the American Psychoanalytic Association*, 48: 1055–1096.
Porges, S.W. (2004) Neuroception. *Zero to Three*, 24 (5): 19–24.
Porges, S.W. (2015) Making the world safe for our children: Down-regulating defense and up-regulating social engagement to "optimise" the human experience. *Children Australia*, 40 (2): 114–123.
Porges, S.W. (2017) *The Pocket Guide to the Polyvagal Theory*. New York: Norton.
Porges, S.W. & Dana, D. (2018) *Clinical Applications of the Polyvagal Theory*. New York: Norton.
Roisman, G.I., Padron, E., Sroufe, L.A., & Egeland, B. (2002) Earned-secure attachment status in retrospect and prospect. *Child Development*, 73 (4): 1204–1219.
Schore, A.N. (2012) *The Science of the Art of Psychotherapy*. New York: Norton.
Siegel, D.J. (2008) *The Neurobiology of "We"* (audiobook). Boulder, CO: Sounds True.
Siegel, D.J. (2010) *The Mindful Therapist*. New York: Norton.
Siegel, D.J. & Hartzell, M. (2003) *Parenting from the Inside Out*. New York: Tarcher.
Stern, D.N. (1985) *The Interpersonal World of the Infant*. New York: Basic Books.
Winnicott, D.W. (1946) Some psychological aspects of juvenile delinquency. In Winnicott, D.W. *The Child and the Outside World*. London: Tavistock, 1957.

9

EMERGENT COMPLEXITY

Freud to neuroscience

Freud's importance to Western culture and sensibility is beyond doubt. As Bloom notes, we can read Freud on anything that troubles us, from envy to fetishism, from mourning to sadism, from love to humor, and we will learn something from that exploration. He has influenced how we read history and psychology and criticize literature. The sheer volume of his writing, his metaphors, and his insights about what it means to be human, continue to enlighten and inform (Bloom, 1986).

So as an icon in European history his place is secure; however, the place of both the theory and technique of psychoanalysis is much less clear and much more endangered. First, his theory has evolved in several different directions, each intellectually important in its own right. These theories both deepen our understanding of our human mind and emotions and also offer contradictory models. Second, his practice of seeing someone five times a week and working through the transference is almost extinct except for training purposes. Surveys reveal that, after training, analysts report seeing fewer than 20 percent of their patients more than once a week, and many of the ones they do see more than once a week are in training (Aron & Starr, 2013). In short, at least in the US, psychoanalysis is not often used as a direct healing modality; rather, it is a complex, useful, in-depth, intellectual understating of the subjectivity of the human mind. It is up to each clinician to use aspects of the insights from the various authors and traditions. As I see it, psychotherapy is the direct healing modality; psychoanalytic thinking is the intellectual underpinnings.

I am interested in ideas out of curiosity but also for the pragmatic reason of, "Can this help me in my life and with my chosen work of practicing psychotherapy?" According to the American Psychological Association, there are more than 200 therapy models but only a few claim to be empirically validated for specific problems. I have already noted several times that, except for Kernberg (2015), psychoanalysis and psychodynamic psychotherapy have not conducted the research that would qualify them as empirically validated.

Big research studies suggest that all effective therapies share four common factors: The first is the client himself and what strengths and support he already has. The second is the quality of the relationship co-created by therapist and client. The hope or expectancy that can be engendered between them is third. And last is the model and the technique associated with that model (Hubble et al., 1999). This book has focused on the last three of these so-called common factors: the model and technique; the relationship; and the idea of optimism, care, and hope. Each client brings his unique qualities, and these are the layers that must be both unpacked and enlivened.

As there are hundreds of forms of psychotherapy, psychoanalysis represents only a tiny fraction of practitioners. Modern therapy of all persuasions must present itself as both helpful and scientifically efficacious. Analysis represents the examined life, the one worth living. Both classical and contemporary psychoanalysis espouse that increased self-awareness will lead to a cessation of symptoms and a higher quality of life. Anyone who has undertaken an analysis or long-term psychotherapy tends to find it life-changing. But has it been proven? It is long and expensive and, as a discipline, it does not present itself well. It has stayed elitist and isolated, typically forming its own institutes away from universities and cross-discipline interactions.

Psychodynamic psychotherapy in the US typically involves meeting weekly and often is conducted face-to-face. Science confirms that human beings orient behavior and expression in response to the face of the other (Ekman, 2003). We all read faces, constantly and unconsciously, in order to create our own sense of self and establish a sense of safety or danger (Porges, 2004). In a therapeutic situation, we especially want to assess the risk of exposing our vulnerabilities to another person. When laying on the couch, we can be more in touch with our inner self without focusing on outside factors. This position encourages reverie and going deeply inside to find oneself. For this reason, there are analysts who place their chair in such a way that, while they can be seen, there is no requirement to stay in face-to-face contact. This can be very useful, especially for patients who are overly compliant and unwilling or unable to move beyond their fear of hurting the other—Brandchaft's pathological accommodation (Brandchaft et al., 2010)

In my mind, today's psychoanalysis divides most clearly over the issue of one-person / two-person as that dictates both theory and technique. The three branches of the British world tend toward one-person and continue to develop theories around drives, the inner world, the developing mind, and the larger human questions inside of each of us. While that style is available in the US, there are many more institutes devoted to the other three branches: intersubjective-, interpersonal-, and attachment-based. All are along a continuum of two-person thinking and deeply interested in the field between analyst and patient, as well as the intrapsychic workings of the patient.

Modern psychiatry is very different. It is strictly biologically based, so both affect dysregulation (the depressive and anxiety disorders) and the psychotic disorders (schizophrenia and bi-polar disorder) are understood as chemical problems that can be best managed with medication. There are hundreds of studies suggesting various levels of efficacy for the drugs needed to help these forms of suffering. There is no doubt medications can help and, in some cases, are critical. However, in most cases, the reality is more nuanced. No drug can help loneliness or create meaning or hope. But they *can* help make meaning, hope, and social connections more possible.

In today's landscape, it is the work of Mark Solms and Karen Kaplan-Solms that stands out as the most rigorous attempt to bring classical psychoanalysis and evidence-based research together. They are steeped in both Freudian psychoanalysis and neuroscience. Both alone and together, they have published a series of books looking at the two disciplines, where they fit together, where they complement each other, and how to look at the brain-mind dilemmas. They use the classical technique of neurology, studying individuals with brain damage through both neuro-imaging and psychoanalysis. They extrapolate from the observed deficits where such mind phenomena as phantasy and dreams reside. Through their cases, they acknowledge the validity of both objective and subjective approaches to the mind.

As scientists, they note that the brain is critical for our survival, mediating between our needs and the dangers and delights of the outside world. Built into our brain are our basic emotion command systems (Panksepp & Biven, 2012), which allow us to respond automatically to important events. Solms reiterates Panksepp's basic systems as key to understanding our brain and, therefore, our mind. He also states that these basic systems, plus the endocrine and reproductive systems, are analogous to Freud's id—that is, these are the body-based motivational systems that unconsciously drive us (Solms & Turnbull, 2002).

For them, the ego begins at the periphery of the body with the sensory end-organs that convey information from the outside world through the spinal cord into the brain itself. Slowly, connections are formed allowing memory to manage impulses, attention, thinking, and judgment. For them, our prefrontal cortex is most closely aligned with Freud's ego (strongly emphasized by Siegel in all of his work). From their neurobiological point of view, the job of all forms of therapy is to strengthen that part of our brain, to give it greater dominion over the unconscious drives of the emotional command systems. They acknowledge that we as yet don't know how it works, but think it requires both language and internalization, the latter artificially rekindled by the unusual safety of the therapeutic tie (Solms & Turnbull, 2002).

The superego also is conceived of as part of the ego system but difficult to localize (Kaplan-Solms & Solms, 2000). Thus, they outline anatomically Freud's structural model. They are appropriately uncertain and humble about these suppositions, presenting them to the analytic community as exciting ideas to start the conversations around neuro-imaging and psychoanalysis.

As I noted above, Solms and Kaplan-Solms write that both the objective knowledge engendered by neuroscience as it studies the brain and its functions, memory, cognition, etc., and the mind as studied by the subjective experience in analysis need to be reconciled. They are two lenses looking at the same mental apparatus.

Jaak Panksepp (1942–2017)

Estonian-born American neuroscientist and psychobiologist Jaak Panksepp (Panksepp & Biven, 2012) documents a useful and complex set of affective drives: seeking, fear, lust, rage, care, panic/grief, and play. He has charted and defined these neural pathways in animal research, and passionately believes that this work needs to be applied to appropriate human research, both for medical solutions and psychotherapeutic interventions.

In our current scientific climate, it is easy to dismiss the subjective. However, for any analyst or therapist, that is not possible. Feelings, memories and imagination are real, although not visible or available for objective study. They are powerful, influence all of our choices and behaviors, and give us the feelings of being real ourselves. Again, Freud was on to something important—albeit, something hard to study and make generalizations about. Currently, neuroscience and psychoanalysis are rather hostile to each other, and Solms and Kaplan-Solms are making a huge effort to create the dialogue necessary to mend that fence. With others, they have created the new discipline of neuropsychoanalysis, which has a journal and a yearly meeting.

I find their work fascinating if a bit difficult to follow since I don't have a strong grounding in brain anatomy. However, like most clinicians, I understand that Broca's area is one of the main locations of language. Kaplan-Solms reports a case of Broca's aphasia, a young man who had suffered a stroke and was almost without words yet was capable of mourning this loss, this disability, using twice-weekly psychoanalytic psychotherapy. One of her conclusions was that, however important that area is to language, it cannot be that important to overall ego functioning, which stayed essentially intact in her work with him. She offers other cases with damage to different parts of the brain where psychoanalysis is not viable even though language is much more accessible (Kaplan-Solms & Solms, 2000).

They also align themselves with Allan Schore's detailed work on understanding the brain relationships to emotions and thinking. However, their close reading of Freud allows them to tie all of their findings directly to his observations; they are much less interested in attachment or any of the more modern, two-person thinking.

Another line of research that is affecting psychoanalysis is that of the various hormonal systems, perhaps part of Freud's id. I have been most interested in the research around oxytocin, which has been proven to be a bonding hormone or a prosocial hormone, as Porges would say. Through animal researchers, such as American biologist and behavioral neurobiologist C. Sue Carter, we have maps of the neurobiology of attachment. Through animal research, she and others suggest that oxytocin bonds mother and baby, and, through human research, we know that it encourages trust and attachment. We know that when the baby is well taken care of, the "care system" comes on line. When the baby is not cared for, the "panic/grief" system is activated (Panksepp & Biven, 2012). We know many of the chemicals that move around those neural nets and are even beginning to make generalizations to distinctly human social emotions, such as compassion (Carter et al., 2017).

Both psychoanalysis and psychodynamic psychotherapy proclaim that we are much more than chemistry, yet they must take the lessons of neuroscience into account to remain viable. For example, at the brain level, the care system and the panic/grief system (Panksepp & Bivens, 2012) constitute the neurobiological substrate of the two sides of what we clinicians call attachment. How can we use this information, integrating it with what is known about developmental trauma from the clinical/subjective side of life?

It is the work of Allan Schore that most robustly combines neuro-imaging techniques, animal research, attachment theory, and psychodynamic psychotherapy. His first premise is that psychotherapeutic change in thinking, without affecting the body-based emotions, is very limited. He calls his work ART, or affect regulation therapy, and aligns it with analysts such as Bromberg (Chapter 7). He is clear that relational trauma in infancy and childhood literally changes the developmental trajectory of the brain towards either a risk for or resilience against later pathology. He documents that psychotherapy changes the brain as well as the mind. Several studies using imaging techniques show that many forms of psychotherapy have physical consequences on the brain (Beauregard, 2014). Schore is very enthusiastic about psychodynamic therapies, as they match his belief that it is only by affecting the "unconscious,"—for him, the right brain—that deep and lasting growth is possible.

On a slightly different but interesting and important angle, we have the seminal studies from Davidson (Davidson et al., 2003) on the brain changes in long-term meditators further boosting the claims for mindfulness and the work of Daniel Siegel.

Other neuroscientists studying the critical space between any two humans, confirming the work of Kohut and Sullivan, include Porges and his polyvagal theory. Specifically, Porges is interested in safety—first physiological and then psychological. He theorizes that our nervous system is designed to anticipate reciprocal interactions and that both psychosomatic symptoms and personality disorders are the result of not getting that interaction. Furthermore, he writes that we are designed for co-regulation beginning with the mother's regulation of her babe. How do we use the Porges (Porges & Dana, 2018) polyvagal theory to understand how devastating the "freeze" response is, and can we learn to unlock its grip? Can we ask similar questions about depression and anxiety? What neurological systems and neuro-chemicals are involved in the creation of a symptom? We really don't know, and we need to know.

For me, the psychoanalytic tradition still represents our deepest understanding of the subjective sense of self, mind, and psyche; our passions, our needs, our dark side, and our self-defeating habits; as well as our longings for connection, wholeness, and creativity. In no way can these be reduced to biology or evolution; at the same time, these underpinnings must be understood and harnessed in the name of therapeutic healing. I trust and hope that analysis continues to evolve, integrating emergent knowledge as it is offered and discarding ideas that are no longer viable. Currently, the neuroscientists I have named are presenting at psychoanalytic conferences, and I take that as a hopeful sign that more developments from that domain will enlarge our capacity to heal the invisible world that Freud first opened up to us.

I have profound respect for this process of walking alongside another human being. All of us have places of inner torment, inner landscapes of guilt and shame, of anxiety, and depression. A practitioner must develop humility and curiosity in order to explore the inner world of another. It is a struggle, requiring courage and heart on both sides. I am amazed that the process that Freud started 150 years ago—without modern imaging equipment or insights from neuroscience—has led us this far. Many devoted people continue this extraordinary undertaking, to both understand ourselves and to relieve the emotional anguish of others. Psychoanalysis, in all of its iterations, creates positive possibilities in the world. Our evolving understanding leads to greater compassion for ourselves and for others, and this must surely enhance all of us in our humanistic endeavors.

The art and science of psychoanalysis now recognizes that the human sense of self or psyche is a very complex, conflicting, and ever-changing process rather than a fixed "something" inside of us. It contains unknowables and cannot be replicated. The study of subjectivity confirms that the self is forever organizing and constantly emerging. Therefore, it is only in the very short term that feelings and behavior can be predicted. The subjective self is non-linear and dynamic, allowing emergent properties to quickly change subjective experience. We are as much indebted to the poets as the scientists as they constantly remind us that life is mysterious and unpredictable. As practitioners we need to hold our ideas lightly and stay present to what is right in front of us.

Early psychoanalysis was based on an essentially linear model of the psyche. The initial view was that once the underlying painful guilt-producing effect is uncovered and faced, change will occur. In this way, Freud and his earliest followers were very optimistic. Sadly, that was not the whole truth of the situation. When we examine life in reverse, we do indeed find a coherence and a set of patterns that make sense. Looking backward, we can see the unhelpful repetitions and the moments of "stuckness" and deadness, and, on the basis of this, we can create a somewhat linear narrative that makes sense to us.

However, when we look forward, we cannot predict what will emerge; we can only set a stage and hope. Psychoanalysis and depth psychotherapy are devoted to creating that safe space—a holding space, a transitional space—where creative exploration can take place in the present moment. Even as we create our best structures to encourage self-reflection and honest sharing, we do not know what will unfold. The process of all psychotherapy is to hold stress and tension in such a way that new growth is possible. We cannot eliminate uncertainty, loss, and emotional pain, but we can hold a space where a client can move between what Siegel (2010) called the poles of chaos and rigidity, overwhelm and deadness. In that process, we hope to find a new and wholesome balance.

Modern psychoanalysis uses the term self and self-states as emergent. Self is neither a thing nor a structure; it is a process. It is constantly created and re-created and requires a constant flow of energy. As therapists, we seek to facilitate this ongoing organic creative process, offering ideas and input, connections, and differing perspectives. We acknowledge that self or psyche is always in relation to different aspects of one's own self, to others, to family, as well as culture—past, present, and future.

It is now clear that the notion of context is critical, especially the context created by relationships. The modern psychoanalyst or psychotherapist seeks to enable self-actualization by creating a safe-yet-not-too-safe context for the therapy (Bromberg, 2011). They want to help their client or patient discover what their most authentic self desires. This is expressed through the way in which that self relates to the analyst in both trust and mistrust. It is presumed that meaning is always co-created between patient and analyst. Our job is to "be" together, not for me, the therapist, to "do" to you, the other.

While the prime contemporary focus is on the affect, the feelings in the moment, we continue to need a narrative. Mary Main's research teaches us that earned secure makes itself known through a coherent narrative (Main, 2000). Schore (2012) and Siegel (2010) both teach that right-brain unknown and unexpressed feelings must be translated into words via the left brain. They, along with Solms and Turnbull (2002), honor the foundation of the brain as well as the much greater complexity of the mind. By strengthening the neocortex and finding words to express ourselves, we gain in capacity to regulate and manage our emotional selves. In attempting to explain a particular human behavior, we create a story, but that story must not be simplistic. "To explain" comes from a Latin root meaning to lay flat, thus potentially creating a "thin" narrative. While we certainly need a story, a narrative line, we must ensure that our understandings are rich, nuanced, and within a context, lest we get caught in a lens of simplistic this-is-the-truth thinking.

Psychological truth is best served by multiple perspectives incorporating complexity, time, and context. We must learn to look at things from different perspectives, simultaneously and without premature resolution. We have to live with paradox, the unknown and unknowable. This can be a source of excitement, possibility, and growth, perhaps even momentary joy and awe, but only if the individual's suffering has subsided sufficiently to tolerate new feelings.

All of the lineages I have laid out currently exist in multiple versions and are taught in many different institutes throughout the US and the UK. They are loosely connected. Self and relational schools of thought especially overlap for American practitioners. Most of these institutes acknowledge the human necessity for reliable contact, for internal coherence, attunement, and the healing cycle of relational disruption and repair. This integration embraces complexity within a system's view of the mind and human relationships. I find that, in current thinking, most of the various disciplines privilege "experience-near," and "heightened affective moments" (Beebe & Lachmann, 2002) and "now moments" (Stern, 2004) as holding the most curative potential. At the same time, they acknowledge the necessity of allowing for multiple points of view and recurrent periods of psychic destabilization. The image of reaching for wholeness while acknowledging its illusive nature captures this contemporary stance. All but the most classical acknowledge ongoing bidirectional influence in all human relationships, fostering a lack of predictability. Not knowing the next step could tip us toward chaos or it might open an unexpected door of new possibility.

Stolorow and Atwood (1992) wrote that theories do not reflect objective realities as much as they do the subjective point of view of their creator. Each theory maker is embedded in his own time and culture as well as in the very issues being discussed. Most modern American analysts, although not all, would agree that a patient's reality is "co-constructed" through the treatment relationship rather than "discovered" through the analyst's objective observation and interpretation.

Circling back to Freud, the game changer, it is clear that his intuition and observations were so very right about many aspects of human subjectivity. His view that we each have a primitive, instinctual inner core; that we are in constant ambivalence and turmoil; and that we have differing parts and points of view remains accurate. His repetition compulsion remains visible in each of us and discouragingly difficult to challenge and undo.

However, Freud's unconscious was a closed system, divided into separate parts by a repression barrier that could be eventually accessed through reflection and words. Today, we acknowledge we certainly do have an unconscious, but it was not created by repression. Rather it is now called the "pre-reflective" unconscious, or implicit knowledge, or sub-symbolic knowing. Anatomically, it is our right brain, our hindbrain and our limbic brain—those parts of our brain that keep us alive and emotionally connected to important others without conscious thought (Siegel, 2010). We now recognize that we cannot access all parts of this system with words. Affective experience is stored mostly in the right hemisphere and the limbic system (Schore, 2012). Neither of these is directly accessible through the reflection and logic of the left brain.

Nevertheless, Freud's very first explanation of what causes psychopathology was right on. Individuals suffering with very debilitating personality disorders have experienced some kind of trauma—have been victimized by emotional, sexual, and/or physical abuse. Milder pathology also is caused by relational trauma, which is the inability of the caring system to meet the real needs of this particular infant. Most modern analysts today agree that pathology is created by the family system's chronic failure to meet the baby's genuine needs, even though they may differ on how to help or heal that failure.

Quickly, Freud came to believe that the inner fantasy life of each infant was much more likely the problem. This was a significant and erroneous shift. In effect, Freud and many of his followers believed that psychological problems were exclusively internal in origin. They might stem from too much innate aggression and its derivatives, such as envy and hate, or too much frustration of the life force, creating unmanageable inner conflicts. This idea still has some credibility. There is no doubt that some infants have more aggression and others exhibit less resilience. Contemporary classical Freudians are more likely to take real trauma into account, but their view as to why an event is traumatizing to some and not others remains linked to personal predispositions, such as innate aggression and vulnerability.

In these schools of thought, the cure still comes from the ability to face and integrate fantasies and impulses.

The question remains: Why do we get so stuck in both our symptoms and our relationships? Each theory and every clinician must seek a particular answer to this specific situation in order to respond to individual emotional pain.

Our first story was Freud's conflict theory: Our psyche is at odds with itself. Within that narrative, we think about drives and impulses and their inhibition, and we work with guilt and anxiety. We assume that development has stopped because the underlying conflict depletes our energy. We believe that freedom will come from becoming aware of and then more able to manage these difficult conflicts. On the other hand, we have come to know that lifting repressions alone may not restart growth. Freud detailed the repetition compulsion and needed to posit a death instinct to account for the difficultly of making a change. In the conflict theory, the central defense is repression, which creates a horizontal split—I don't want to know these parts of me, it would be too painful, too shaming, too destabilizing.

With "Gail," it was immediately apparent to me that she was unconsciously jealous of her adult daughter. She wanted a better relationship with her daughter, and the daughter was a recurring theme during our time together. Gail's story was that the daughter was disrespectful and distant. Gail felt judged by her daughter and reported that she felt like a victim, but she could not contact what she felt in her body as we talked. Both of us found it difficult to track and explore the flashes of sadness and anger that animated her face for brief moments. After many months of weekly contact, Gail was able to follow her anger at her daughter in the present moment and discover how jealous she was of the daughter: her youth, her opportunities, and her marriage. Gail found it difficult to face what she judged as unkindness in herself. Her shame was great. She believed that, in feeling her jealousy, she was eradicating her genuine love for her daughter. We worked to help her hold both as true. She was jealous, and she also loved. More conscious of the jealousy, Gail was able to see her part in the daughter's disrespect. By understanding how she and her daughter trigger one another, she was able to move out of a simple cause-and-effect narrative—"My daughter was disrespectful to me"—into a more complex picture involving words, facial expressions, and tones of voice continually occurring between two people.

The current story held strongly by the self psychology lineage and those involved in the attachment lineage is that of arrested development. Normal psychological growth has been impeded by some kind of family or environmental failure. This is currently referred to as "relational" or "strain" or "environmental" or "developmental" trauma. Something missing or thwarted in childhood leads to deficits in adulthood. When we work with this idea, we know that insight *per se* will not lift the suffering. The client must have a different lived experience within the therapy, an emotional experience. Guntrip (1969) was one of the first to realize and write about this perspective on psychological pain. In accordance with this belief, therapy must revitalize stalled developmental strivings and encourage the mourning of what never was and perhaps can never be.

In the developmental arrest story, the major defense is dissociation, or a vertical split, meaning there are parts of the self rendered inaccessible, in cold storage. This suggests multiple self-organizations and multiple self-states that truly do not know each other (Bromberg, 2011). Working with a vertical split to revitalize and connect split off parts is never easy and always involves both a "real" relationship as well as the transference relationship.

A third useful theory is the emerging research on affect regulation. In this narrative, the disorganizer is terror—terror of separation and abandonment, which stops energetic flow and makes connecting with others difficult if not impossible. Panksepp is clear: Terror is *not* fear intensified. Fear activates the fight/flight response. We know from animal research that fear and panic travel on different neural pathways. Terror is extreme panic. Terror is the panic of any young mammal separated from and/or threatened by its significant other. Terror activates the freeze reaction, which is a biological-psychological response that lies deeper in the nervous system than fight and flight. Freezing is always beyond choice, and it invariably inhibits learning on any level. When in a state of panic or terror, nothing new is possible—no learning, no nuances, no possibilities (Panksepp & Biven, 2012).

Dissociation in response to terror represents an interpersonal event that has been internalized, forming the core of extremely disruptive trauma. My story of Ruth is one of both arrested development—as an adult, she operated more like an abused child, vulnerable both at home and at work—and that of being hijacked by the feeling of terror, leaving her unable to stay in the present with a real, caring other. In such cases, the present slips and falls into an unconscious landscape of former relationships. The same can be said of Jack, who jumps between his own rage and terror in seconds as if his parent's unpredictable rage was in the room right now.

All of these theories are lenses on the truth of complex subjective reality. With experience, most clinicians will flow seamlessly among them, intuiting when to help the other face his own demons, when to acknowledge the terror of traumatic dissociations, when to focus on understanding the past, and when to stay strictly in the present moment—the "between" of analyst and patient.

Many studies suggest that the analyst's theory of pathology and change is less important than his or her ability to make a connection—attachment, again—with the patient (Hubble et al., 1999). What allows for change? The classical model leans towards interpretation, moving slowly, confronting and uncovering more and more psychic layers. The cure for the suffering comes from heightened self-awareness. And it is certainly true that being listened to and emotionally understood is healing in and of itself. The Christian theologian Dietrich Bonhoeffer (1954) wrote, "Often a person can be helped merely by having someone who will listen to him seriously . . . we should listen with the ears of God." Good advice to any therapist of any persuasion.

Freud intended psychoanalysis to be empirical, a natural science, conducted in some variety of a laboratory setting. The analyst was to be objective, offering silent listening and, occasionally, a correct interpretation. The patient's response was proof that, with a correct interpretation, repression could be lifted, and an ongoing sense of self could be restored. This stance is now referred to as one-person psychology, where the analyst believes he can act on the patient from a clear, separate place of wisdom and well meaning.

In this classical form, the meeting is the medium through which the mental contents inside of the patient become known. All that occurs happens because of the patient and his past. Working with the transference from this perspective means that the unacceptable feelings of "there and then"—wanting to murder, exploit, merge—are felt now with the analyst and within the analytic setting. The job of the objective analyst is to open the door to these repressed, unacceptable feelings and then help the patient integrate these into his ongoing sense of self.

Done well, this classical form has real strengths. Most practitioners are devoted to their patients, care deeply about their inner life, respect the subjectivity of the other, and know that we all carry the same basic humanity. They understand that attention and deep listening heal. The creation of the frame—coming at the same time to the same room and working within agreed boundaries—provides a sense of being attended to and held. Although they would not use the metaphor, this work is a right-brain-to-right-brain process of deep personal connection. On the other hand, this stance of strict neutrality within classical analysis can enable some analysts to stay distant, less uninvolved, and "hidden behind the couch," leaving the patient feeling very alone and isolated.

Currently, many more analysts and therapists work within the two-person psychology model. Here, the change agent is not only the safety of the relationship, but also life-giving involvement and reanimation provided by deeply felt emotions. These feelings can occur when the analyst/therapist acknowledges they are as embedded in the situation as the patient, bringing awareness of their own conflicts and needs to the therapeutic encounter. This analyst/therapist acknowledges, at least internally, that they too, are looking for validation and connection. The interaction creates meaning for both, albeit in different ways. Acknowledging that the therapist/analyst brings their past into the consulting room means that the neutral observer is no longer a possibility.

This interactional model requires that both parties stay in the present, co-created moment as much as possible. This analyst assumes that both are using what has been learned from their separate pasts to weave this unique relationship in the present. This model offers interpretations and questions, suggesting feelings and attitudes come from the patient's past. However, the patient's experience of the analyst is no longer only a total displacement from the past. It will always have some truth in it; something happened in the present to alert the patient that he was in danger, or misunderstood, or ignored, or not seen or valued. By taking the stance that both parties are contributing to the moment, the analyst can acknowledge his part in the relationship while also confirming the patient's view of reality.

However, there also is the implicit message that the analyst is different from those figures of the past. This change of model implies that, in therapy, growth and change become possible when the patient has different lived experiences with this new "other," allowing him to develop new and better attitudes toward himself, his significant others, and his overall life. The analyst offers some form of the basic, parental responsiveness that was missed (Bacall, 1985), alleviating negative feelings, shame and "stuckness," allowing development to proceed in a more creative, flexible way.

Currently, some schools of thought hold that the therapist must offer reliable attention, careful listening, and thoughtful interpretations that arise from being in reverie. These are believed to be enough to reanimate development. Others think the therapist must offer more—more availability and/or responding more positively than the patient's parents. Such schools maintain that the analyst must show real caring and gratify some of the patient's desires in some subtle way in order to create the necessary attachment and avoid further re-traumatization. Most schools assume there are two levels operating all the time: the parent–child line of history and the adult–adult line of the present (Bacall, 1985).

The inner world of the analyst was once called "specific countertransference," and for Freud and his followers, it was important to uncover one's feelings about each patient and neutralize them. It was assumed that the analyst's own feelings could be kept out of the room through a proper personal analysis. It was believed that providing evenly hovering attention would bring up only the patient's issues, leaving the analyst out of the equation. Things were seen to have gone off course if the analyst was triggered into reactive emotions during the session. This could only mean that the analyst's past was intruding into the present.

But following first Sullivan and Fromm and currently Stern, Schore, and Siegel, most now believe that the mind is an interactive field between two people. We each evoke different responses from one another all the time, and the analyst needs to value his personal reactions as containing useful information about the patient, himself, and the interaction. Contemporary thought suggests that the patient's repetitive interpersonal difficulties will have an effect on the analyst. And the analyst, as a person, will in turn have a direct energetic effect on the patient. These bodily felt responses occurring in the therapist/analyst are now considered a vehicle for moving the process forward for the benefit of the patient.

In a fully two-person system, both analysts and therapists know they have vulnerabilities and that eventually all patients will get under their skin in some way or another, evoking personal responses (Mitchell, 1997). When we care and are deeply engaged, we will be affected. Most analysts now view themselves as vulnerable human beings rather than objective observers or reflecting mirrors. Each of us has a different professional stance in line with our training and our personality. We all know that how we dress, the look of our office, and what we choose to reveal or not reveal communicate who we are in fundamental ways. Patients pick up information through their senses in the same way we do. For example, imagine the experience of a patient whose analyst arrives in the waiting room from the outside world after the patient has taken a seat there. Compare this to the feeling of finding the analyst there, waiting for him when he arrives. This may never be spoken of, but certainly it will have been registered somewhere in the patient's being.

Some analysts encourage their patients to share what they see and experience in the analyst, both to encourage the patient's trust in his own perceptions and to engender the idea of "theory of mind," where each party has a mind and can make educated guesses at what is going on in the other's mind. Other analysts do not ask for such information directly, assuming that what is important will arise in the conversations over time.

One thorny issue is that of personal disclosure. In the classical model, it was clear: Disclose nothing of yourself, see everything in the room as belonging to the patient. The contemporary Kernberg is explicit that total nondisclosure is an essential condition for the patient to feel free enough to explore his own fantasies (Mitchell & Black, 1995). If the analyst gives himself permission to disclose, it might foreclose deeper introspection, according to Kernberg's way of thinking. Other schools use some disclosure (Aron, 1996; Bromberg, 2011) as long as the focus is both in the present moment and on the client's experience: What does it mean to the client? In his writings, Bromberg reports that he often discloses what he is thinking in the present moment about the patient and their interaction. He is certainly not talking about confessions or defensive explanations to ward off anger or even misunderstanding. Used well, many have found that some form of disclosure can be useful, enhancing authenticity and a collaborative spirit. One of the theoretical foundations for some disclosure is that it permits the creation of new object relationships. An analyst may need to be quite active for a frozen, dissociated traumatized patient to feel any human mutuality: *If you have feelings about me, I matter to you! If you have feelings about me, perhaps I am real, I exist.*

In *A Meeting of Minds*, Aron (1996) discusses at great length the confusing issue of self-disclosure. He notes that overall self-revelation is inevitable, so the real issue is when and how does the analyst deliberately self-disclose. The relationship is in continuous negotiation, like every human relationship. I am most interested in his observations around the paradoxical aspects of the therapeutic relationship. It is both intimate and spontaneous, yet professional, even technical. It must be authentic yet focus on the patient. Money is exchanged. How does that influence the power and responsibility? Aron gives us as many questions as answers.

Each analyst–patient dyad must create the optimal bond and degree of disclosure in order for the patient to feel seen and valued. As a psychologist, I regularly refer to psychiatrists when I think that medication might be helpful. I think about what qualities in that other professional might help create a bond with my patient. One discloses her family needs when she is making appointments—*I don't work late on Thursdays, as I have to get my daughter to ballet.* For some of my patients, that is reassuring. It shows that she is "a person like me" with a life and distractions. For others, it indicates she is "unprofessional" and probably not very attentive to her patients, as she is too focused on her children. It is not a matter of a right or wrong way of being; rather, it is what works for the person in need, and that it can be talked about and emotionally explored.

Modern-day psychoanalysis is both on the wane as a technique and intellectually vividly alive. Various institutes are offering everything from in-depth classical training to courses online for diplomas in depth psychotherapy. Their conferences are often a source of great intellectual rigor and excitement, covering everything from gender issues to aging, from the exploration of an individual case to generalizations about war, political psychopathology, and compassion. To explore the world of psychoanalysis is to enter a world of both compassion and rigorous conceptual analysis on some of our thorniest issues. Like the current conception of the self, it is continuously exciting and renewing for psychotherapists of all persuasions.

Key concepts Chapter 9

Affect regulation theory – our normal human need is to connect with others and manage our own feelings; this can be disorganized by terror, stopping energetic flow, making connecting with others difficult

Arrested development – normal biological and psychological growth has been impeded by environmental failure

Conflict theory – Freud's first understanding of human motivation, observing that our psyche is at odds with itself

Countertransference – the feelings the analyst has about the patient. In one-person psychology these must be managed through the analyst's personal analysis, keeping the analyst neutral. In two-person psychology these feelings are used as data about this specific relationship

Dissociation – a "vertical split," meaning there are parts of the self rendered inaccessible to awareness; the consequence of terror or trauma of any kind

Healing cycle – involves relational disruption and repair

One-person psychology – stance that each of us in maturity is solid and separate within our skin; in contrast to two-person psychology which suggests that we are all affecting each other all the time

Personal disclosure – what, if anything, to reveal to the patient about oneself as the therapist in the service of healing

Postmodern psychoanalysis – recognizes that the human sense of self or psyche is very complex and contradictory, and that healing requires both theoretical knowledge and a strong interpersonal connection

Psychological truth – is not a simple narrative and is best served by multiple perspectives incorporating complexity, time, and context

Safe space – a holding space, a transitional space—where creative exploration can take place and therapy is possible

Self – currently thought of as an emergent property. It is neither a thing nor a structure; it is an ongoing process derived within a context

Terror – biological-psychological response deep in the nervous system that is beyond fear and choice; Panksepp's panic circuit

Two-person psychology – the idea that the change agent is the safety of the therapeutic relationship and that emotions flow in both directions; real care is necessary to provide reanimation and transformation

Unconscious – today, referred to as pre-reflective unconscious rather than Freud's repressed unconscious and thought to be in the implicit nonverbal right brain and subcortical regions of the brain

References

Aron, L. (1996) *A Meeting of Minds*. Hillsdale, NJ: Analytic Press

Aron, L. & Starr, K. (2013) *A Psychotherapy for the People*. New York: Routledge.

Bacall, H. (1985) Optimal responsiveness and the therapeutic process. In Bacall, H. (ed.) *Optimal Responsiveness*. Northvale, NJ: Jason Aronson, 1988.

Beauregard, M. (2014) Functional neuroimaging studies of the effect of psychotherapy. *Dialogues in Clinical Neuroscience*, 16 (1): 75–81.

Beebe, B. & Lachmann, F.M. (2002) *Infant Research and Adult Treatment*. Hillsdale, NJ: Analytic Press.

Bloom, H. (1986) Freud, the greatest modern writer. *New York Times Book Review*, March 23, pp. 1, 26–27.

Bonhoeffer, D. (1954) *Life Together: The Classic Exploration of Christian Community*. New York: Harper & Row.

Brandchaft, B., Doctors, S., & Sorter, D. (2010) *Towards an Emancipatory Psychoanalysis*. New York: Routledge.

Bromberg, P.M. (2011) *The Shadow of the Tsunami*. New York: Routledge.

Carter, C.S., Bartal, I.B.A., & Porges, E.C. (2017). The roots of compassion: An evolutionary and neurobiological perspective. In Seppala, E.M. et al. (eds) *The Oxford Handbook of Compassion Science*. New York: Oxford University Press.

Davidson, R.J., Kabat-Zinn, J., Schumacher, J., Rosenkranz, M., Muller, D., & Santorellie, S.F. (2003) Alternations in brain and immune function produced by mindfulness meditation. *Psychosomatic Medicine*, 65: 564–570.

Ekman, P. (2003) *Emotions Revealed*. New York: Times Books.

Guntrip, H. (1969) *Schizoid Phenomena, Object Relations and the Self*. New York: Basic Books.

Hubble, M.A., Duncan, B.L., & Miller, S.D. eds. (1999) *The Heart and Soul of Change*. Washington, DC: American Psychological Association.

Kaplan-Solms, K. & Solms, M. (2000) *Clinical Studies in Neuro-psychoanalysis: Introduction to a Depth Neuropsychology*. New York: Karnac.

Kernberg, O. (2015) Resistances and progress in developing a research framework in psychoanalytic institutes. *Psychoanalytic Inquiry*, 35: 98–114.

Main, M. (2000) The Adult Attachment Interview: Fear, attention, safety and discourse process. *Journal of the American Psychoanalytic Association*, 48: 1055–1096.

Mitchell, S.A. (1997) *Influence and Autonomy in Psychoanalysis*. Hillsdale, NJ: Analytic Press.

Mitchell, S. & Black, M. (1995) *Freud and Beyond*. New York: Basic Books.
Panksepp, J. & Biven, L. (2012) *The Archaeology of Mind*. New York: Norton.
Porges, S.W. (2004) Neuroception. *Zero to Three*, 24 (5): 19–24.
Porges, S.W. & Dana, D. (2018) *Clinical Applications of the Polyvagal Theory*. New York: Norton.
Schore, A.N. (2012) *The Science of the Art of Psychotherapy*. New York: Norton.
Siegel, D.J. (2010) *The Mindful Therapist*. New York: Norton.
Solms, M. & Turnbull, O. (2002) *The Brain and the Inner World*. New York: Other Press.
Stern, D.N. (2004) *The Present Moment in Psychotherapy and Everyday Life*. New York: Norton.
Stolorow, R.D. & Atwood, G.E. (1992) *Contexts of Being: The Intersubjective Foundations of Psychological Life*. Hillsdale, NJ: Analytic Pres.

GLOSSARY

A

Abandonment or separation anxiety the intense panic experienced when separated from the mother for too long; now considered the source of much psychological suffering in adults

Active questioning Sullivan's technique to understand and help heal his patients; in distinction to the classical "blank screen" analyst

Adult Attachment Inventory the structured interview devised by Main to determine an adult's attachment style; used extensively by Siegel in his work integrating psychotherapy and mindfulness

Affect dysregulation the state of being unable to manage one's feelings or thoughts

Affect regulation refers to the universal need to manage both feelings and thoughts to maintain inner continuity

Affect regulation theory our normal human need is to connect with others and manage our own feelings; this can be disorganized by terror, stopping energetic flow, making connecting with others difficult

Affect regulator a current term for talking about how important others are to each of us in maintaining emotional well-being, both to soothe and to enliven

Affectivity one of Stern's core qualities, the capacity to feel feelings

Agency one of Stern's core qualities, the capacity to act on one's own behalf

Alpha elements Bion's idea that the baby's first primitive thoughts must be transformed into alpha elements through interaction with a more mature mind

Ambivalent attachment style an insecure style involving both clinging to and rejecting others

Anaclitic depression the normal emotional response of grief and anger of a child who is separated from his caring others for three months or less

Anxiety the feeling of not being safe

Area of creation Balint's term for the first months of life, wherein the babe is self-contained and full of potential

Arrested development normal biological and psychological growth has been impeded by environmental failure

Attachment theory Bowlby's assertion that the infant needs consistent care in order to develop physically and psychologically

Autistic-contiguous mode Ogden's contribution to the Kleinian positions; refers to a sensory, bodily mode of being that underlies her two modes of experiencing

Avoidant attachment style an insecure style that involves keeping a large emotional distance from significant others

B

Bad objects refers to people or aspects of people who have been incorporated into the psyche as negative, unpleasant, or even endangering

Basic fault Balint's term for the early time of life where the world is naturally split into good and bad moments due to the care and failure of care the babe receives. With too much failure of care, the babe does not develop psychically beyond this phase

Benign regression refers to Balint's belief that the patient needs to regress to a state of trusting dependency on the analyst in order to start over

Beta elements refers to Bion's conceptualization of the baby's first way of thinking

Bion's theory of thinking the babe's beta elements, our earliest way of thinking is gradually transformed into alpha elements through interaction with another, more mature mind. Never considered "real," rather a way of thinking about thinking.

Body-ego the idea that ego functioning is based in the sensations and experiences of the physical body; first put forth by Freud

Borderline a personality disorder involving splitting both the self and others into discrete good and bad aspects; emotionally very unstable and painful

C

Capacity for concern as the babe develops, according to Winnicott, she becomes aware that others exist, and she can care about them and affect them

Castration anxiety what the little boy fears in the fantasy of excluding his father in order to have an exclusive relationship with his mother

Central ego Fairbairn's term for the conscious aspect of the original ego that is stripped of vitality

Classic psychoanalytic technique the analytic stance of neutrality, listening carefully, offering a few interpretations from an out-of-sight position

Co-determined a modern assumption that relationships including analytic relationships involve emotional, nonverbal, and verbal input from all parties

Cohesion one of Stern's core qualities, the capacity to experience oneself as whole

Collecting impingements a pattern of relating that assumes others will not treat me well, thereby creating that exact experience

Conflict theory Freud's first understanding of human motivation, observing that our psyche is at odds with itself

Contained Bion's metaphor alluding to the baby's emotional/physiological needs in which beta upsets are transformed into alpha states

Container Bion's metaphor for the mother's ability to manage her baby's upsets

Core sense of self Stern's phrase for the baby's development when his emergent senses of self are mirrored and allowed to flourish

Countertransference the feelings the analyst has about the patient. In one-person psychology these must be managed through the analyst's personal analysis, keeping the analyst neutral. In two-person psychology, these feelings are used as data about this specific relationship

Cycle of rupture and repair Beebe and Lachmann's description of the pattern between mother and baby of attuning, misattuning, distress and repair of that distress

D

Death instinct a Freudian hypothesis to explain our destructive and self-destructive aspects

Defense mechanisms include projection, regression, sublimation, reaction formation, undoing, reversal, introjection, turning against the self

Defenses the patterns each of us creates in order to avoid psychic pain and vulnerability

Depressive position one of Klein's basic positions wherein the infant is able to hold both aspects of self and mother, the good, and the bad

Despair profound grief, hopelessness, and helplessness; for a baby if separation from the "care-er" is too long, the infant gives up and retreats into himself with a darkened mood

Destiny drive Bollas' belief that each of us wants to thrive and wants to find the best environment to experience our personal essence

Detachment the creation of a defense or false self to manage the pain of inappropriate separation; the final step of the separation cycle

Developmental arrest within self psychology, pathology is created when the basic needs of a developing infant are not met and growth is curtailed

Developmental deficits the consequence of stalled development due to poor care in early childhood resulting in missing resiliency or ego strength

Developmental tilt Mitchell's stance that too often analysis privileges early childhood history over present-day interactions to the detriment of self-responsibility and growth

Developmental or strain trauma when a parent does not meet a baby's needs in a timely and appropriate fashion the infant suffers; when this happens a lot, the infant's very sense of self is formed around the sense of not being taken care of, thus traumatized

Dismissive attachment avoidant attachment in adults, keeping emotional distance

Disorganized/dysregulated attachment when the caregiver evokes fear rather than safety the baby lives in a terrified state not able to find safety with others or within himself

Dissociation a "vertical split," meaning there are parts of the self rendered inaccessible to awareness; the consequence of terror or trauma of any kind

Drive-conflict model according to Freud, sexuality and aggression are basic to instinctual life and they need discharge either in fantasy or literally, creating conflict with others

Dynamic structures Fairbairn's theoretical understanding of how the baby gathers his sense of self at the very beginning of life through undergoing "good" and "bad" experiences with his caregivers

Dysregulation refers to the human capacity to feel not whole, integrated, or good when thoughts and feelings run out of control; usually need another to regulate and provide safety and soothing

E

Earned secure Main's observation that some adults transform an insecure style of attachment to a more secure style through positive life experiences

Ego in the structural model of id, ego, and superego, the ego is the mediator between the drives of the id and the superego ideals of the family and culture

Ego ideal a fantasy created by the growing self of how I should be or wish to be; always unrealistic, but important as a human striving

Ego psychology one of the branches to evolve which privileges the ego and ego strength over the more primitive drives of the original Freudian theory

Ego strength the capacity of the ego or self (depending on the psychoanalytic school) to manage both inner impulses and needs as well as outer stressors

Eight stages of man Erikson's outline of growth and development throughout the life cycle

Emancipatory therapy Brandchaft's theory and practice of analysis that emphasizes pathological accommodation and existential freedom

Emergent the process of coming into being, specifically the human mind and sense of self as processes, rather than fixed structures

Emergent sense of self Stern's research, based on observations that each infant contains the capacity for agency, affectivity, cohesion, and self-history

Empathic immersion Kohut's analytic technique encouraging the analyst to see the world through the needs and feelings of his patient; a subjective stance

Empathy our inbuilt capacity to emotionally understand others and therefore to connect with them. An important curative term in the lexicon of self psychology

Enactments inevitable behaviors that take place between analyst and patient that are created by unconscious frozen patterns that need to be "translated" into words and insight

Environmental mother at the beginning of life the baby experiences the environment as dedicated to meeting his needs, not a person who takes care of him

Eros Freud's term for the positive life force including sexuality and sensuality

Exciting object Fairbairn's term for that aspect of the mother that satisfies and frustrates the baby; sometimes referred to as the frustrating exciting object

F

Face for Levinas, the face holds an ethical call to offer the "other" infinite compassion and care

False self Winnicott's term for defensive structures designed to protect the true self from further harm or impingements

Fear of freedom Fromm's position that we fear fully being ourselves and instead comply to the wishes and demands of others in order to keep their love and connection

Frame the conscious agreements between analyst/therapist and patient including time and money

Free association the invitation to speak whatever comes to mind without censoring

Frustrating mother in object relations, that aspect of the mother that does not meet every need of her baby in a timely fashion

G

Generativity Erikson's term for the best of adult development, the capacity to create, find meaning, and give back

Going-on-being Winnicott's idea that the well cared-for baby experiences few impingements so as to feel herself as alive, continuous, and content

Good enough mother she is not perfect or rigid, yet holds her baby and his needs in mind most of the time and is willing to fulfill those needs

Greed wanting more than the other can give; one of Klein's core qualities of the newborn

Guilt is explained by both the Oedipal theory and the gaps between the superego ideals and the ego's ability to live up to those ideals

Guilty man Freud's Oedipal theory is built on guilt as the driver in distinction to Kohut's tragic man who is searching for connection and meaning

H

Harmonious interpenetrating mix-up Balint's phrase for the ideal relationship between mother and babe; it is effortless and reciprocal

Hartmann's ego adaptation the belief that the ego can constantly create and adapt to new situations

Hatching Mahler's phrase noting that the baby emerges gradually from her felt experience of being at one with the mother and begins the separation-individuation journey

Healing cycle involves relational disruption and repair.

Hermeneutics a term in philosophy and later psychoanalysis describing the science of interpretation, noting that the lens we use for interpreting others determines what follows

Hermeneutics of suspicion Orange's term for the classical Freudian lens; things are not as they appear to be

Hermeneutics of trust Orange's term for the lens humanistic psychology and some others employ when sitting with patients; the patient will unfold in her own time when provided with safety and care

Hospitalism the apathy or failure to thrive a child falls into when separated for too long from those he needs and depends on

Hysteria historically referred to a collection of vague, unaccountable symptoms, such as excessive emotionality, attention-seeking behavior, and bouts of amnesia, found exclusively in women

I

Id in the structural model of id, ego, and superego, the id is the basic driver of unconscious, instinctual life

Idealize to hold in high regard; specifically, for Kohut the need children have to see their parents as good so that they can internalize those strengths and capabilities

Idealized other the baby's implicit appraisal of the people he is dependent on, his objects, paired with the central ego

Idealizing transference Kohut's belief that it is important for many patients to idealize their analyst in order to incorporate new positive aspects

Impingements anything that disrupts going-on-being

Incorporate and expel good and bad objects object-relations language for how the baby internalizes aspects of his caretakers

Individuation process the normal growth pattern of decreasing dependence on the caring others as the excitement of exploration develops

Insecure attachment the dynamic created when the caretaker can't meet enough of the baby's needs; the baby cannot rest in safety

Internal saboteur or sadistic superego that aspect of the self formed in relation to the rejecting object

Internal working model Bowlby's term for the baby's unconscious understanding of the relationship between himself and his "care-er"

Interpersonal space Sullivan's focus for treatment, less inside the other and more in the space between two living human beings

Intersubjective field a further development of self psychology that conceives of the analytic relationship as composed of the space between two subjects working together on behalf of the patient

Intersubjectivity the complex field of interaction between analyst and patient creating emotional connection as opposed to a subject and object of study

I–thou Buber's injunction that we treat each "other" as a sacred, important being; he also realized it was an ideal

K

Kleinian positions idea that from the very beginning the babe can both "split" the world into good and bad and integrate the world into a more whole sense of you and me within the container of the mother

L

Latent content what the dream is pointing to after being understood in a deeper, richer way using both free associations and interpretations

Libidinal ego that aspect of self formed in relation to the exciting object

Libidinal object the good each baby both creates and discovers in his caring other

Libido the energy of Eros and sexuality

Lived emotional experience both Balint and Guntrip emphasized that patients need a real relationship with a real other in order to have a new emotional experience

Love affair with the world Mahler's phrase for the joy expressed by the infant as he learns to walk and explore; usually around the end of the first year of life

Love made angry and love made hungry Guntrip's description of the baby's possibilities when his needs are not met

M

Malignant regression Balint's observation that some patients get stuck in dependency, and do not move towards mourning and new beginnings

Manic defense developed capacity to override painful feelings through action, discussed in great detail by both Klein and Winnicott

Manifest content the images and narrative remembered from a dream

Marking the facial gestures a caregiver makes to help her baby distinguish between his emotional state and hers as first noted by Fonagy

Me–not me the baby's first boundary in the development of self

Mentalization-based treatment Fonagy's therapy to help people who suffer from disorganized attachment issues to regulate their feelings and thoughts

Middle or independent school the group of analysts who did not side with either Anna Freud or Melanie Klein, who insisted that the infant was object-seeking, not drive discharge-seeking and that the relationship with the analyst needed to involve care

Mid-life depression Erikson noted that many people suffered a loss of meaning and depressed affect when they had accomplished their material or conscious goals

Milieu therapy using inpatient settings, Sullivan created a healing environment involving every aspect of living

Mindfulness a spiritual practice that has been modified to incorporate it into psychotherapy to manage anxiety, reduce stress, and heighten awareness; a core technique in Siegel's work

Mirror a first basic need of the baby that his inner life, his feelings be mirrored by the face, tone, and sounds of the mother

Mirroring transference a basic need of a patient to have his emotions reflected back to him by the analyst thus validating the reality and necessity of those emotions

N

Narcissism a term used to describe a continuum of characteristics from healthy agency to pathological self-centeredness

Narcissistic rage rage that stems from feeling intense humiliation; it includes the need to destroy the cause of that humiliation

Negation saying the opposite of what is true; a Freudian defense

Neo-Freudian schools of thought that have derived from Freud, but modified both theory and technique

Negative transference experiencing the analyst/therapist in an automatically negative light

Neurotic level a developmental achievement post-psychotic level, wherein anxiety is managed through various defenses

Neutralization Hartmann's concept that the ego could reduce the power of the id drives, rather than sublimate or re-direct that power, as Freud proposed

Normal autistic phase Mahler's first phase of development; later renamed as her research demonstrated that the neonate is always relational, never self-contained

Normal symbiotic phase Mahler's term for the second stage of development during which the baby is believed to experience himself as often merged with the mother or caring other

O

Object refers to the people who care for the baby allowing him to incorporate them or parts of them into his sense of self

Object mother the "real" or personal mother who cares for this specific baby

Object-relations theory an in-depth understanding of mental life as based on the infant's first experiences with others, specifically family

Objective love and hate the idea that there are aspects of patients that warrant strong approval and strong disapproval, but that offering such direct feedback must be carefully titrated into a useful interpretation

Oedipal complex a developmental stage wherein the young child desires an exclusive relationship with the parent of the opposite sex and fears retribution from the parent of the same sex

One-person psychology stance that each of us in maturity is solid and separate within our skin; in contrast to two-person psychology which suggests that we are all affecting each other all the time

P

Paranoid-schizoid position one of the two basic Klein positions wherein the infant splits the world into good and bad, both sense of self and the other

Participant observation an analytic stance that acknowledges the analyst's contribution to the relationship; at the same time the analyst and patient are not equals, the analyst keeps an appropriate distance monitoring the transaction

Part-objects Klein's understanding that at the beginning the baby can relate to a part of a person—for example, just the breast

Pathological accommodation Brandchaft's theory that unconscious compliant attachment is a major source of both pathology and suffering

Personal disclosure what, if anything, to reveal to the patient about oneself as the therapist in the service of healing

Phantasy Kleinian understanding of how the built-in drives of the babe are elaborated through unconscious experience early in life

Play according to Winnicott, in health, play for a child is the simple ability to enjoy and dramatize her inner life; for an adult it is the capacity to use language and other symbols to express the true self without rigidity or anxiety

Positive transference experiencing the analyst/therapist in an automatically positive, even idealized, light

Postmodern psychoanalysis recognizes that the human sense of self or psyche is very complex and contradictory, and that healing requires both theoretical knowledge and a strong interpersonal connection

Practicing phase part of Mahler's developmental model when the babe is consolidating physical movement, at around one year

Pre-moral at the beginning of life, the baby is not concerned with right and wrong; she is concerned with survival. Concern and morality are developmental achievements within a caring context

Pre-Oedipal issues the inner dynamics created at the very beginning of life when the baby's experience is discontinuous in time allowing him to exist as if both he and his mother could be all good and wonderful or all bad and beyond terrible

Preoccupied attachment ambivalent attachment in adults

Primary love the first object relationship between the babe and her mother

Primary maternal preoccupation the state of being of "ordinary" mothers who are focused primarily on their newborns

Projection a Freudian defense, whereby an aspect of self is disowned and given to another to carry

Projective identification first understanding of primitive bodily communication; how feelings from one person get into another before language

Protest an essential part of the cycle of attachment and separation

Psychological truth is not a simple narrative and is best served by multiple perspectives incorporating complexity, time, and context

Psychology of the self Kohut's theories as distinct from Freud's drive theory

Psychotic level a universal aspect of the human mind that exists before rational thought and the ability to manage emotional distress

R

Rapprochement phase Mahler's term when the two-year-old discovers the conflict between his desire to be separate and his desire to be connected

Real relationship in distinction to the transference relationship. Both are ongoing and the "real" relationship is especially important in dealing with pre-Oedipal issues

Reciprocal mutual influence Hartmann's idea that the baby and the mother are affecting each other and need each other continually; important to both self psychology and relational psychology

Rejecting object Fairbairn's term for that aspect of the mother that frustrates the babe too much of the time

Relational psychoanalysis the analytic school evolving from the work of Sullivan that emphasizes the importance of both real and imagined relationships from the beginning of life as the cause of emotional pathology

Relational trauma also referred to as "strain" trauma; when the parent does not attune to and mirror the child, the child develops a set of defenses to survive, foreclosing the possibility of spontaneous, joyful living

Relational-conflict model Mitchell's understanding that the patient needs both a new relationship and a willingness to be confronted in difficult ways

Repetition compulsion our capacity to endlessly repeat a traumatic or distressing pattern over and over in dreams and/or behavior

Repression one of Freud's basic defenses: our human capacity to put painful emotions or experiences out of awareness

Reverie refers to first the mother's and then the therapist's ability to understand what is going on inside the other through using his own inner life

Right brain to right brain Schore's understanding that emotional connection and communication happen through the right side of the brain, nonverbally and unconsciously in both babies and adults. It is the location of effective psychotherapy

Ruth–ruthless at the beginning of life, the babe demands that her needs be met immediately—Winnicott referred to this early stage as ruthless and that over time, she develops "ruth"

S

Sadistic super ego see internal saboteur

Safe space a holding space, a transitional space—where creative exploration can take place and therapy is possible

Safe surprise Bromberg's phrase for the best way to bring a new and perhaps challenging idea or insight into a patient's awareness

Schizoid factors Fairbairn's term for psychic development when needs are not met, and the babe depends too much on his inner fantasies to meet his real needs

Secure attachment knowing that the "care-er is reliable and dependable creating inner safety

Secure base attachment theory's understanding that the external caregiver creates safety and the capacity to thrive in an infant; over time that safety is internalized into an inner secure base

Selective inattention Sullivan's phrase for how a child separates himself from his mother's anxiety

Self currently thought of as an emergent property. It is neither a thing nor a structure; it is an ongoing process derived within a context

Self psychology the analytic school of Kohut, noting that the struggle to be valued emotionally and understood first by family, then by others, creates meaning and growth throughout life

Self-actualization our innate capacity to psychologically grow and develop

Self-object Kohut's term for any person who is used to help create a sense of self; self-objects are needed throughout life in order to thrive

Self-states Bromberg's acknowledgment that within each of us reside many different "selves," and sometimes these inner states are not overlapping or aware of each other

Separation anxiety the fundamental source of all anxiety—away from the secure base and safety

Separation-individuation phase with mobility, the toddler begins to explore her world still needing the secure base of the mother

Separation-individuation theory Mahler's developmental theory based on direct observations of mother–child pairs

Shame a felt sense of diminishment and deficit, a sense of falling from grace and wholeness; increasingly a focus of clinical work

Significant other Sullivan's observation that we need special people in our lives, starting with our first caregiver

Social engagement system Porges' designation of the human preference to gaze at another face, make eye contact, hear the human voice, and gesture to communicate

Split world at the beginning, the babe does not live in linear time, so each experience is discrete, creating a "good mother who takes care of me" paired with a "wonderful me" and a "bad mother who does not" paired with a "frustrated me"

Splitting at the beginning of life when the baby does not live in time it is normal to experience the world as split into good and bad moments; this becomes a pathological stance if there has been too much deprivation, and healthy ambivalence cannot emerge

Spontaneous gestures of emotional creativity Winnicott's phrase for the natural aliveness within each human being; it is a goal of therapy to restore access to that aliveness

Strange situation the laboratory experiment devised by Ainsworth to determine attachment style

Structural model the interplay of the id, ego, and superego—psychic structures hypothesized by Freud to explain what he was experiencing as an analyst

Subjective sense of self as development proceeds, the infant gathers enough of a self to recognize that he and another are different or separate

Superego in the structural model of id, ego, and superego, the superego holds the ideals and the injunctions from parents and culture

Survival both mothers with their baby and therapists with their patient need to "survive" negative experiences with neither retaliation nor withdrawal, coming to experience one another as two separate people

T

Terror biological-psychological response deep in the nervous system that is beyond fear and choice—Panksepp's panic circuit

Thanatos the death instinct, including our self-destructive tendencies

Theory of mind the innate ability to know I have thoughts and feelings and you have thoughts and feelings and when around you I have some idea of your state of being. Was first a philosophical stance and is now a concept researched by developmental psychology

Topographical model the idea that the conscious is but a small part of our psychic structure and the unconscious is much larger and more in control than we imagine

Tragic man Kohut found that psychoanalysis needed to create meaning, in distinction to Freud who found that psychoanalysis needed to relieve the suffering of guilt

Transference Freud noticed and named the fact that our first experiences as infants unconsciously shape how we relate to others in the future, especially important others or figures in authority

Transformational object Bollas' characterization of the mother as one who transforms the baby's internal and external environment by managing his psychosomatic needs

Transitional objects soft objects that soothe the baby, reminding him of his mother and her care; they both connect him to her and allow the process of separation

Transitional space a space that is co-created by mother and babe, by analyst and patient, where change is possible. It is a dimension of living that is neither external nor internal; rather it is both

True self / false self Winnicott's radical proposal that each individual contained a true self that would never disappear even though it could go into cold storage and be hidden by one or more false selves

Twinship transference Kohut's belief that some patients need to see themselves as "like" their analysts and therefore as positive

Two-person psychology the idea that the change agent is the safety of the therapeutic relationship and that emotions flow in both directions; real care is necessary to provide reanimation and transformation

U

Unconscious today, referred to as pre-reflective unconscious rather than Freud's repressed unconscious and thought to be in the implicit nonverbal right brain and subcortical regions of the brain

Unthought known Bollas' phrase for the unconscious source of actions and behavior, derived from interacting with others in early life and never thought about

V

Vicarious introspection the form of empathy Kohut believed would allow the patient to feel understood and valued

W

Wish fulfillment originally, the idea that a dream was pointing to what the dreamer truly wanted

Working alliance the phrase the ego psychologists used to describe the relationship between analyst and patient

INDEX

abandonment anxiety 57, 71, 99, 129–130, 134, 156
abdication 51
Abraham, Karl 22
Abram, J. 74
abuse 7, 66, 113
accommodation 96, 128
activation 129
active participation 117
active questioning 108–109, 115
adaptive development 53, 55
adolescence 50, 132
Adult Attachment Interview 133–134
affect regulation 82, 119, 137, 138–139, 156
affect regulation therapy (ART) 151
affective drives 150
affectivity 98, 99
agency 33, 53, 60, 74, 80, 92, 98, 117
aggressive impulses: Erikson, Erik 60; Freud, Anna 51; Freud, Sigmund 6, 8, 12, 15, 16, 17, 49; Kernberg, Otto 41, 42; Klein, Melanie 27, 32–33, 37; Kohut, Heinz 91, 93; and narcissism 93
Ainsworth, Mary 3, 55, 131–132, 134
alienation 89, 112
alpha elements 38
alter ego 92
ambivalent attachment 130, 132, 133, 134
American Journal of Psychiatry 110
American Psychiatric Association 110
American psychoanalysis: overview of 23, 24, 148; and Anna Freud 52; Aron, Lewis 115–116; Beebe and Lachman 99–101; Bowlby, John 3; Brandchaft, Bernard 95–98; Bromberg, Philip 119–121; ego psychologists 49; Erikson, Erik 58–61; Fromm, Erich 111–112; Hartmann, Heinz 52–54; Kernberg, Otto 41–43; Kohut, Heinz 88–93; Mahler, Margaret 56–58; Main, Mary 133–135; Mitchell, Stephen 116–119; modern models of psychotherapy 148; Ogden, Thomas 43–46; Spitz, René 54–56; Sullivan, Harry Stack 107–111; Thompson, Clara 112–113; United States schools of psychology 3
American Psychological Association 147
anaclitic depression 55
anal drive 15, 17, 27
analysts analyzing each other 27, 52, 69, 77, 79, 113
anger 36, 41, 55, 58, 78, 80, 91, 128, 130, 155
Anna Freud National Centre for Children and Families 135
anti-libidinal object relationships 66
anti-medication approaches 83
anxieties 80, 108, 109, 117, 148
apprentice model of training 24
area of creation 69
Aron, Lewis 3, 114, 115–116, 147, 159
arrested development 79, 90, 93, 95, 100, 110, 117, 155–156
art and culture 53, 75
'as if' self 89
asymmetrical relationships 103, 115, 121, 159

attachment 3, 23, 96, 118, 125–132, 148, 150, 151, 155, 156, 158
attunement 10, 12, 44, 74, 99, 100, 102, 137, 138, 140–141, 143, 153
Atwood, George 3, 93–95, 154
authentic self 112
authenticity 93, 118, 159
authoritarian relationships 111
autistic-contiguous mode of experiencing 44–45, 56, 69, 98
automation conformity 111
autonomy 15, 58, 59, 74, 90, 111, 118, 134
avoidant attachment 130, 132, 133

babies, infants and early development: Atwood and Stolorow 95; Balint, Michael 69; Bollas, Christopher 81–82; Bowlby, John 125–130; Fairbairn, Ronald 65–66, 67; Freud, Anna 52; Freud, Sigmund 8, 15; Guntrip, Harry 79; Hartmann, Heinz 53; Klein, Melanie 26–27, 28, 29–30; Mahler, Margaret 56–58; Spitz, René 54–56; Stern, Daniel 98; Sullivan, Harry Stack 109–110; Winnicott, Donald 73–74; *see also* developmental theory; mother-infant relationships
Bacall, H. 158
bad objects 28
Balint, Michael 3, 23, 68–72, 75, 81, 130
Balint Groups 72
basic assumptions 102
basic fault 69, 71
basic trust 59, 71, 118
Bateson, G. 94
beating fantasies 49
Beauregard, M. 151
Beebe, Beatrice 3, 99–101, 135, 137, 153
being with 64, 93, 103
benign regression 71
Bergman, Anni 56
beta elements 38, 44
biological creatures, humans as 4–5, 125
biological givens 98
Bion, Wilfred 3, 37–40, 45–46
bi-polar disorder 148
Biven, L. 149, 150, 151, 156
Black, M. 9, 16, 22, 27, 28, 29, 30, 31, 32, 33, 35, 39, 40, 41, 42, 52, 55, 59, 61, 67, 74, 93, 108, 109, 110, 112, 116, 117
Bleandonu, G. 37, 38, 45
Bloom, Harold 4, 5, 147
body-ego 44
body-mind separation 5
Bollas, Christopher 3, 81–83
Bonhoeffer, Dietrich 156
borderline personality difficulties 41, 42, 58, 93
boundaries of the self 67, 95
Bowlby, John 3, 21, 23, 125–130, 135
brain structures 138, 140, 149, 150, 151, 153, 154; *see also* neuroscience
Brandchaft, Bernard 3, 95–98, 128, 148
breakdown, fear of 78
breaking the link 39
breasts 26–27, 28, 33, 74
Brenner, C. 9, 27
Bretherton, I. 126, 130, 131
Breuer, Josef 6
British middle school 2, 3, 23, 64–87
British Psychoanalytical Society 65
Broca's area 150
Bromberg, Philip 3, 54, 118, 119–121, 129, 132, 151, 153, 156
Buber, Martin 1, 102, 103, 121, 141
Budapest 69, 113
Budapest Society 27
Burlingham, Dorothy 50

calling, analysis as a 79
capacity for concern 74
caregiver relationship 125; *see also* mother-infant relationships
Carter, C. Sue 150
castration anxiety 16
central ego 67
character analysis 49
Charcot, Jean-Martin 6
Chicago Institute for Psychoanalysis 88
children: analysts analyzing own 22, 27, 48; Freud, Anna 50; Freud, Sigmund 15; Klein, Melanie 27; Winnicott, Donald 72–78; *see also* babies, infants and early development; developmental theory; mother-infant relationships
classic technique 13–14, 23, 53, 64, 77, 91, 108, 115, 157
clinical supervision 24, 119
closure 95
co-creation 46, 95, 100–102, 114, 115, 140, 148, 153, 154
co-determination 96
cognitive behavioral methods 43
coherence 92, 152, 153
cohesion 98
collaboration, therapy as 118, 159
collecting impingements 75–76, 97

communication: mother-infant communication 36, 99–100; nonverbal communication 36, 39, 101, 103, 128, 129, 136, 138, 143; projective identification 36; unconscious interpersonal communication 101, 138, 141
companion, therapist as 130
compassion 139, 140, 150
compliance 76, 97, 128, 134
conflict and adaptive development 53
conflict anxiety 99
conflict theory 8–9, 155
conformity 111
connection, need for: Balint, Michael 70; Brandchaft, Bernard 96, 97; Buber, Martin 102–103; Freud, Sigmund 8, 10, 13; Fromm, Erich 111, 112; Kernberg, Otto 42; Klein, Melanie 32; Kohut, Heinz 90, 93; Main, Mary 135; Mitchell, Stephen 118; in the psychoanalytic tradition 151; Schore, Allan 138; Spitz, René 55; Stern, Daniel 98, 99; Sullivan, Harry Stack 109, 111
container ↔ contained 38, 44
contextualism 23, 74, 92, 93, 153
cooperative groups 140
co-participation 114
core sense of self 98–99
co-regulation 151
cortisol 127
countertransference 43, 76, 94, 95, 101, 158
creativity 75, 76, 90, 92, 93, 96, 111, 135
cycle of rupture and repair 100, 101, 137, 153

Dana, D. 151
Darwin, Charles 4, 8
Davidson, R.J. 140, 151
death instinct 8, 91, 155
defenses: analysts' (in modern relational psychoanalysis) 114; dissociation 7, 37, 119, 142, 156; false selves 73; Freud, Anna 49; Freud, Sigmund 12, 13–14; Kernberg, Otto 42; and language 108–109; manic defense 32; projective identification 35–37, 39, 101
dehumanization 103
delinquency 118, 127
denial 51
dependency 52, 57–58, 70, 71, 79, 90, 134
depression 28, 51, 59–62, 80, 129, 148
depressive anxieties 80
depressive positions 27, 31–32, 35, 44
deprived childhoods 50, 54
depth psychotherapy 17, 152, 160
despair 8, 32, 59, 67, 79, 81, 90, 92, 97, 126
destiny drives 82–83
detachment 126–127
developmental arrest 79, 90, 93, 95, 100, 110, 117, 155–156
developmental deficits 23
developmental theory: adaptive development 53, 55; adulthood 59–60; Ainsworth, Mary 131; attachment theory 125–143; Bowlby, John 127; Bromberg, Philip 119; Erikson, Erik 59–60, 118; Fairbairn, Ronald 66; Freud, Anna 50, 52; Freud, Sigmund 8–9, 15–16, 17, 27; Guntrip, Harry 79; Hartmann, Heinz 53; individuation process 28, 57, 70, 73, 112, 118, 119, 128; Kernberg, Otto 41; Klein, Melanie 22, 30, 31; Kohut, Heinz 89–90, 92, 93; Mitchell, Stephen 118; separation-individuation theory 56–58; Spitz, René 54–55; Sullivan, Harry Stack 109–110; Winnicott, Donald 74, 78
developmental tilt 117–118
developmental trauma 54, 119–121, 151, 155
dismissive attachment styles 134
disorganized attachment 130, 132, 133
dissociation 7, 37, 119, 142, 156
dissociative identity disorder 132
doctor-patient relationship (primary-care physicians) 72
dreams 14–15, 78
dreams, unrealized 92
drive theories: and the ego psychologists 53; Erikson, Erik 59; Fairbairn, Ronald 65; Freud, Anna 52; Freud, Sigmund 3, 8–9, 155; Hartmann, Heinz 53; Kernberg, Otto 41; Klein, Melanie 26–27, 28; Sullivan's alternative to 111
dynamic structures 66–67
dysregulation 119, 129, 130, 132, 139, 148–149

each other, analysts analyzing 27, 52, 69, 77, 79, 113
earned secure attachment 135
edge 118
ego: Bromberg, Philip 121; Fairbairn, Ronald 65–66, 67; Freud, Anna 49; Freud, Sigmund 9, 17; Kohut, Heinz 92; and neuroscience 149, 150; and projection 35
ego adaptation 52–54, 55
ego ideal 9

ego integrity 59
ego psychologists: beginnings of 2; Brandchaft, Bernard 95–98; Erikson, Erik 58–61; Freud, Anna 22, 48–52; Freud's lineage 3; Hartmann, Heinz 52–54; Kernberg, Otto 41; Klein, Melanie 22; Mahler, Margaret 56–58; Spitz, René 54–56; and the traditional father figure 71
ego roots 53
ego strengths 51, 80
Einstein, Albert 8
Ekman, P. 101, 138, 148
emancipatory therapy 97
emergent senses of self 98, 152
empathic immersion 23, 89, 91, 93, 94, 97, 117
empathy: and the British middle school 64; Erikson, Erik 61; Kernberg, Otto 42; Klein, Melanie 31, 32; Kohut, Heinz 23, 89, 90–91, 93; and mentalization 136; Stern, Daniel 99
enactments 36, 98, 114
enlivened vitality 100
enlivening others 73
environmental mother 75
envy 32–35, 42, 54, 60, 73
Erikson, Erik 3, 58–61, 118
Eros 8, 27
ethics 102, 103
ethnology 23, 125
evacuees 72, 126
evidence-based practices 43, 56, 135–136, 147, 149
evolution 8
examined life 14, 148
exciting objects 66
experience-near 153

face 103
face-to-face interactions 103, 148
failure to thrive 55
Fairbairn, Ronald 3, 23, 27, 65–68, 71, 73, 80
false selves 73, 76, 97, 127
family therapy 94
fantasy: Fairbairn, Ronald 67; Freud, Sigmund 7, 8; Hartmann, Heinz 53; hope as 118; Klein, Melanie 29; Kohut, Heinz 91; and phantasy 29; Winnicott, Donald 78
father figures 71
fathers 37
fear of freedom 112
feminism 113
Ferenczi, Sándor 21–22, 69, 113
fight/flight response 30, 138, 142, 156
Fonagy, Peter 3, 23, 128, 129, 132, 135–136
formative years 17, 18; *see also* babies, infants and early development; developmental theory
fragmentation of self 22
frame, therapeutic 11–12, 103, 114, 121–122, 157
free association 7, 9, 13, 49
free will 111
freedom 111, 112
freeze/faint response 142, 151, 156
Freud, Anna 48–52; and the British middle school 64; ego psychologists 22; and Fairbairn 68; and Freud's lineage 3, 5, 17; and Heinz Kohut 90; and London 21, 50
Freud, Sigmund 4–20; body-ego 44; and the British middle school 64; classic technique 13–14, 23, 53, 77; desire to create objective natural science 2, 4–5, 8–9, 83, 157; developmental theory 15, 17; dreams 14–15; drive-conflict model 8–9, 17; and Erich Fromm 111; exclusive concern with internal psyche 126, 154; guilty man 90; and Harry Stack Sullivan 108; hermeneutics of suspicion 102; on hope 118; later theory 17–18; lineage 3, 18, 21, 147; mourning 17; and neuroscience 149; Oedipal complex 16; primary process thinking 65; resistance 97; secondary process thinking 53; technique 9–14; trauma 6–7; and the unconscious as a closed system 154; and World War I 8, 24
Freud, Sophie 18
Freudian slips 5
Fromm, Erich 3, 158
frustrating exciting object ↔ libidinal ego 66

Geller, S.M. 142
generativity 59, 60
genetics 138
genital drive 15
Gerhardt, S. 127, 128, 129, 132, 133, 138
going-on-being 73, 82, 143
Goleman, D. 140
Gomez, L. 65, 67, 69, 70, 72, 80
good enough mother 74–75, 78, 81, 91, 139, 140–141
good life 111, 112; *see also* meaningful life
grandiosity 89, 91
gratification 28, 53, 71, 118

greed 32, 34–35, 42
Greenson, R.R. 13, 60, 61
grief 17, 52, 129, 150
Grosskurth, P. 22, 27, 28, 30, 64
Grotstein, J.S. 37, 38, 40
guilt 16, 31, 32, 35, 80, 91, 119, 152
guilty man 90
Guntrip, Harry 3, 23, 27, 77, 78–81, 155–156

Hampstead Clinic 50
hands, holding 71, 77
harmonious interpenetrating mix-up 69, 70, 81
Hartmann, Heinz 3, 52–54
Hartzell, M. 133, 134, 135, 140
hate 31, 32–35, 41, 42, 60, 73, 76–77
healing cycle 100–101, 137, 153
heightened affective moments 153
Herman, J. 7, 65
hermeneutics 102
hierarchy of needs 110
history (biological given) 98
holding environments 74, 152
Holmes, J. 126
Holocaust 93, 102
home base, secure 91
honesty 112
hope 59, 118, 127, 148, 149, 152
hopelessness 33, 67, 81
hormonal systems 150
hospitalism 55, 126
Hubble, M.A. 148, 156
humanism 93, 111, 112, 116, 130
humiliation 33
hysteria 6–7

id: Bromberg, Philip 121; Freud, Anna 49; Freud, Sigmund 8, 9, 15, 17; Hartmann, Heinz 53; and hormones 150; and neuroscience 149; Spitz, René 55; Winnicott, Donald 73
ideal objects 67
idealized other 29, 42, 90, 91, 95
idealizing transference 92
identification 49
identity crisis 59
imagination 7, 8, 29, 67, 126, 136–137
immediate gratification 28
impingements 75–76, 97
incest 7, 27
individuation process 28, 57, 70, 73, 112, 118, 119, 128
inner boundaries 95
instinctual drives 12
integrated individuals 9, 12
integrating tendencies 109
intention 73, 101, 129
interdependencies 70, 79, 118
internal working model 128–129
internalization 9, 59, 66, 92, 96, 111, 127, 136, 149
interpersonal neurobiology 137–139, 143
interpersonal relationship psychoanalysis 107–124; Aron, Lewis 115–116; beginnings of 23; Bromberg, Philip 119–121; Fairbairn, Ronald 65; Ferenczi, Sándor 22; Freud's lineage 3; Fromm, Erich 111–112; Mitchell, Stephen 116–119; and modern psychoanalysis 148; and psychiatry 110; Stern, Daniel 99; Sullivan, Harry Stack 107–111; Thompson, Clara 112–113
intersubjectivity: Aron, Lewis 115; Atwood and Stolorow 93–95; Bowlby, John 129; Brandchaft, Bernard 95–98; intersubjective thinking 101; Kohut, Heinz 90; and modern psychoanalysis 148; Ogden, Thomas 45
intimacy 13, 35, 42, 57, 59, 70, 90, 115, 121, 129, 159; *see also* connection, need for
introjection 34, 49
introspection 78, 89, 90
introspective-empathic method 90–91
intuition 140
invisible, coming to understand the 5
irritating actions 97
isolation 59, 89, 93, 107, 111, 112, 136; *see also* loneliness
I-thou 102–103, 121, 141

jealousy 33
Jewish heritage 24, 41, 102
joy 82–83, 90
Jung, Carl 21–22

Kaplan, L. 57
Kaplan-Solms, Karen 149, 150
Karen, R. 127, 129, 130, 131, 134
Kernberg, Otto 3, 41–43, 45–46, 93, 102, 147, 159
kindness 140
Klein, J. 41, 66, 67, 69, 70, 79, 80, 81
Klein, Melanie 26–37; and the British middle school 64; ego psychologists 22; exclusive concern with internal psyche 126; and Fairbairn 68; and Freud's lineage 3; hermeneutics of suspicion 102; lineage 2, 45–46; in London 21,

22, 26, 27; positions 30–32, 44, 49, 54, 58, 65; primitive agonies 27; and Winnicott 72, 73–74
Kohut, Heinz 2, 3, 23, 88–93, 97, 100, 117, 118, 137, 151

laboratory research 131, 142
Lachmann, Frank 3, 99–101, 153
Langs, R. 11
language use 108–109, 122, 136, 149, 150, 153
latency period 50
latent content of dreams 15
learning from mistakes 100
Levinas, Emmanuel 102–103
Lewis, Thomas 135
libidinal ego 66
libidinal objects 55
libido: and aggression 51; Fairbairn, Ronald 66; Freud, Anna 49, 51; Freud, Sigmund 8, 17, 53; Klein, Melanie 27, 30, 37; Spitz, René 55
linear models of the psyche 152
Little, Margaret 77, 78
lived experience 65–66, 114, 122, 136–137, 138, 158
London 21, 26, 27, 50, 65, 131, 135
loneliness 108, 109, 111, 112, 135, 136, 149
longitudinal studies 131, 133
loss 129–130
love: Atwood and Stolorow 95; Balint, Michael 69–70, 71; Bion, Wilfred 41; Erikson, Erik 59; Fairbairn, Ronald 66, 67; Fonagy, Peter 137; Freud, Sigmund 90; Fromm, Erich 111; Guntrip, Harry 79, 80, 81; Hartmann, Heinz 53; Kernberg, Otto 42; Klein, Melanie 31, 35, 37; philosophy 102; primary love 69–70, 71; Spitz, René 55; Winnicott, Donald 74, 76–77, 78

Mahler, Margaret 3, 56–58, 99
Main, Mary 3, 132, 153
malignant regression 71
manic defense 32
manifest content of dreams 15
marking 137
masculine as assumed standard 27
Maslow, Abraham 1
Masterson, J.F. 58
meaningful life 83, 93, 102, 149
medicalization of suffering 101, 148
meditation 151
melancholia 17
memories 6–7, 12–13, 28, 149
me–not me 41, 42, 44, 79, 81, 119
mentalization 135–136
mentoring 74
merger 42, 79, 81, 130
metaphoric partnerships 61
metaphors 61
metaphysical concepts of humanity 59
micro-tracking experiments 100–101
mid-life depression 59–62
milieu therapy 109
mindfulness 23, 139–141, 151
mirroring 74, 75, 77, 79, 91, 117, 119, 134, 137
mirroring transference 92, 95
misattunement 100
Mitchell, Stephen 3, 9, 16, 22, 27, 28, 29, 30, 31, 32, 33, 35, 39, 40, 41, 42, 52, 55, 59, 61, 67, 74, 93, 102, 108, 109, 110, 112, 115, 116–119, 158
morality 76, 79, 135, 138, 140
Morrison, A.P. 92
mother figure, analyst as 71
mother-infant relationships: Ainsworth, Mary 131–132; Aron, Lewis 115; attachment 3, 23, 96, 118, 125–132, 148, 150, 151, 155, 156, 158; Balint, Michael 69; Beebe and Lachman 99–101; Bion, Wilfred 38; Bollas, Christopher 82; Bowlby, John 126, 128–129; Fairbairn, Ronald 65–67; Fonagy, Peter 136; Fromm, Erich 111–112; good enough mother 74–75, 78, 81, 91, 139, 140–141; Hartmann, Heinz 53; Klein, Melanie 28, 36, 37; Main, Mary 133; Ogden, Thomas 44; Porges, Stephen 151; separation-individuation theory 56–57; Spitz, René 55; Stern, Daniel 98–99; Sullivan, Harry Stack 109; Winnicott, Donald 74–75
motor development 57, 128
mourning 17, 31, 52, 92, 95, 129
mutual vulnerability 116
mysticism 37

narcissism: Kernberg, Otto 41, 42, 93; Kohut, Heinz 23, 89, 90, 91–92; separation-individuation theory 58; and shame 92
narcissistic rage 91, 97
narratives 153
negation 12, 102
negative emotions 28, 32–35, 73
negative transference 11, 13
neocortex 138, 153
neo-Freudians 23, 58

nervous system 142, 151
neural nets 150
neurobiology 137–139, 150
neurochemicals 102, 127, 151, 154
neuroplasticity 60, 139
neuropsychoanalysis 150
neuropsychology 137–139
neuroscience 18, 23, 29, 45, 81, 82, 119, 127, 132, 138, 140–143, 149–151, 153
neurosis 5, 12, 15, 41, 42
neutrality, of analyst: Beebe and Lachman 101; Bion, Wilfred 40; classic technique 13–14, 23, 157; early American psychotherapy 108; Freud, Anna 48; Freud, Sigmund 11, 12, 13, 22, 23; Fromm, Erich 112; Guntrip, Harry 78, 79; Kernberg, Otto 43; modern relational psychoanalysis 114
neutralization 53
non-duality 37–38, 40
nonverbal communication 36, 39, 101, 103, 128, 129, 136, 138, 143
now moments 153

object mother 75
objective hate 77
objective love 77
objectivity, scientific 2, 4–5, 8–9, 83, 95, 149, 157
object-relations theory: and the British middle school 64; Fairbairn, Ronald 65; Freud, Anna 52; Guntrip, Harry 79; Kernberg, Otto 41–42; Klein, Melanie 22, 28, 29, 32; Ogden, Thomas 45
Oedipal issues 16, 17, 37, 41, 50, 69, 90
Ogden, Thomas 3, 43–46, 98
omnipotence 74, 89
one-person psychology: Aron, Lewis 115; Erikson, Erik 61; Freud, Sigmund 157; Kernberg, Otto 43; Klein, Melanie 36; Kohut, Heinz 93; and modern psychoanalysis 148; Ogden, Thomas 46; Winnicott, Donald 74, 78
open-ended inquiry 115
opposites, holding 39
oral drive 15, 17, 27
Orange, Donna 3, 12, 101–103
orphanages 54–55
others, need for 65–66; *see also* connection, need for; loneliness
oxytocin 150

panic/grief systems 150, 151
Panksepp, Jaak 149, 150, 151, 156
paradox as part of the human condition 44
paranoid-schizoid position 30–31, 32, 41, 44, 58
parasympathetic nervous system 142
partial selves 66
participant observation 109, 112, 113, 114, 121
part-objects 27, 28
pathological accommodation 96–98, 100, 128, 148
patient ↔ analyst 39, 40
peak experiences 1
Perry, H.S. 23, 108, 109, 110
personal disclosures 103, 159
personality disorders 132, 154
phallic drive 17, 27
phantasy 28, 29, 35, 65, 66, 70, 149
Phillips, A. 78
philosophy 101–103
physical contact, analyst-patient 12, 71, 77
physiological effects of separation 127, 129
Pine, Fred 56
play 31, 75, 76
play therapy 26
pleasure-seeking drive 9, 12, 15, 27, 41, 53, 55
political psychology 111
polyvagal theory 142, 151
Porges, Stephen 3, 138, 142–143, 148, 150, 151
positions, Kleinian 30–32, 44, 49, 54, 58, 65
positive transference 10–11, 14
post-Oedipal development 50
potential space 75
poverty 107, 108
prefrontal cortex 140, 149
premature sexuality 6, 7
pre-moral stages 79
preoccupied attachment styles 134
pre-Oedipal issues 22, 27, 79
pre-reflective unconscious 154
present, focus on the 112, 113, 115, 116, 117, 118–119, 157
pre-subjective experience 99
pre-symbolic experience 44
primary love 69–70, 71
primary maternal preoccupation 74
primitive agonies 27, 29
primitive nature 8, 17
professional groups 72
projection 35, 49, 71
projective identification 35–37, 39, 101
protest 126, 128, 130, 131
psychiatry 5, 24, 83, 101, 108, 110, 148–149, 159
Psychoanalytic Dialogues 115

Psychoanalytic Institute, Vienna 21–22
psychobiology 150
psychosis 37, 39, 41, 42, 83, 107, 108, 148
psychosocial development 59
PTSD (post-traumatic stress disorder) 6, 37, 65

rage 30, 31, 32, 43, 44, 45, 67, 91, 156
rapprochement phase 57, 58, 99
reaction formation 49
real relationship 79, 97, 156
reciprocal mutual influence 94
reconstruction versus interpretation 90
regressed ego 80–81
regression 39, 43, 49, 58, 71
regret 31, 32
rejecting object ↔ sadistic superego 67
relational school 107–124; Aron, Lewis 115–116; beginnings of 3, 23, 103; Bromberg, Philip 119–121; compared to neuropsychology 141; Fromm, Erich 111–112; and Jung 22; Mitchell, Stephen 116–119; Sullivan, Harry Stack 107–111; Thompson, Clara 112–113
relational trauma 97, 98, 151, 154
relational-conflict model 118
reparation 28, 32, 35, 91, 100, 137
repetition compulsion 12–13, 118, 155
representational models 128–129
repression 7, 12–13, 17, 119, 154
research: Ainsworth, Mary 131; Ekman, Paul 101; evidence-based practices 43, 56, 135–136, 147, 149; Fonagy, Peter 135–136, 137; Freud, Anna 50, 52; longitudinal studies 131, 133; Mahler, Margaret 56; Main, Mary 133; neuroscience 148, 149, 151; Spitz, René 54–55; Stern, Daniel 98–99
resilience 52, 61, 91, 151
resistance 97
re-traumatization 97, 158
revenge 97, 127
reverie 38, 68, 148, 158
reversal 49
risk taking, encouraging 120
Riviere, Joan 22, 27, 28, 31, 32, 35
Rodman, F.R. 22
Rogers, Carl 1
Roisman, G.I. 135
root causes, finding 6
Ruesch, J. 94
rupture and repair, cycle of 100, 101, 137, 153
ruth/ruthlessness 74

sadism 67
safe surprise 120
safety 49, 66, 73, 75, 76, 91, 113, 118, 120, 127, 138, 149, 151, 153
schizoid factors 55, 67–68, 79, 80, 81, 83
schizophrenia 108, 148
Schore, Allan 3, 129, 137–139, 141, 150, 151, 153, 158
Scotland 65, 68
secondary process thinking 53
secure base 126, 128
security operations 114; *see also* defenses
Segal, H. 27, 29, 31, 34
selective inattention 110
self, sense of 41, 66, 70, 91, 98, 138, 140, 141, 143
self ↔ selfobject 92
self fragmentation 79, 90, 92
self psychology: Atwood and Stolorow 93–95; beginnings of 3, 23; Brandchaft, Bernard 95–98; compared to neuropsychology 141; compared to relational 115, 117–118; Freud's lineage 3; Kohut, Heinz 88–93
self-actualization 1
self-analysis 14, 49–50
self-awareness 31
self-care 77
self-continuity 143
self-destruction 33
self-disclosure 103, 159
self-esteem 33, 52, 108, 128, 134
self-harm 43
self-hate 34, 35, 43, 80, 97
self-object 90
self-object boundaries 41
selfobjects 90, 92
self-states 121, 152–153, 156
sensory experience 44
separation anxiety 57, 67, 99, 126–127, 130, 131–132, 133, 156
separation-individuation theory 56–58
sexual abuse 7
sexuality 8–9, 15, 16, 42, 111
shame 91–92, 120
sibling groups 50–51
Siegel, Daniel 3, 60, 89, 133, 134, 135, 138, 139–141, 149, 151, 152, 154, 158
social engagement 142
social psychology 111
social recovery 109
Solms, Mark 149, 150, 153
Solnit, A. 50
spirituality 60
Spitz, René 3, 54–56, 126

split world 29, 30, 41, 42
splitting 67, 119, 155, 156
spontaneity 76, 79
stagnation 59
Starr, K. 115, 116, 147
statistical analysis 131, 133
Stern, Daniel 3, 98–99, 135, 140, 153, 158
still-face experiments 100
Stolorow, Robert 3, 93–95, 154
Storr, A. 13, 15
Strachey, James 22
strange situation 131
strengths and gifts, focus on 90, 148
Strozier, C.B. 23, 88, 90, 93
structural model (Freud) 17
subjectivity: analyst as meaning-making 117; and the British middle school 64; and modern psychoanalysis 150, 152; and neuroscience 149; subjective sense of self 98–99; Winnicott, Donald 75, 77; *see also* intersubjectivity
sublimation 49, 53
Sullivan, Harry Stack 2, 3, 23, 107–111, 115, 151, 158
superego 9, 17, 49, 149
supportive professional groups 72
suspicion, hermeneutics of 102
symbiotic phase 56–57
symbolic thinking 31
symmetry 102
sympathetic nervous system 142
systems theory 94, 95

terror 156
Thanatos 8, 27
theory of mind 129, 130, 136–137, 159
therapeutic frame 11–12
Thompson, Clara 3, 112–113, 115
three-person system 69, 83
topographical model 17
tragic man 90, 92
training of analysts 24, 49, 65, 72, 78
transcendent position 38, 40
transference: ego psychologists 60–61; Freud, Anna 51; Freud, Sigmund 7, 10–11, 17; Kernberg, Otto 42, 43; Kohut, Heinz 92; and neuroscience 147, 156, 157; versus reciprocal mutual influence 94
transference-focused psychotherapy 42, 43
transformational objects 82–83
transitional objects 75
transitional space 75
trauma: analysts' own 28; and delinquency 127; developmental trauma 54, 119–121, 151, 155; and dissociation 142; in early years 79, 90, 119–121, 154; Freud, Sigmund 6–7; Guntrip, Harry 79; and personality disorder 154; and regression 71; relational trauma 97, 98, 142, 151, 154; re-traumatization 97, 158; and transitional objects 75; traumatic loss 95; and war 24, 65
traumatic memory 7
Tronick, Edward 100
true self 73, 74, 75, 76, 82, 97, 121
trust 38, 51, 59, 70, 71, 73, 78, 91, 102, 118, 134, 135, 153
truth 40, 121, 153
Turnbull, O. 149, 153
twinning 91, 92, 95
two-person theory: Aron, Lewis 115; Bion, Wilfred 40; Brandchaft, Bernard 96–97; modern mindfulness 141; and modern psychoanalysis 83, 103, 148, 154, 157–158; modern relational psychoanalysis 114; Ogden, Thomas 45

Uganda 131
unacceptable self 17
unconditional positive regard 1
unconscious: and brain structure 138; destiny drives 82–83; and dreams 15; ego and superego 9; fantasy 53; Freud, Sigmund 12, 13, 154; Fromm, Erich 112; id 8; interpersonal communication 101, 138, 141; mother-infant communication 99–100; pre-reflective unconscious 154; projective identification 35–37; reverie 38; Schore, Allan 151; social creation of 112; true and false selves 73; unthought known 81–82
undoing 49, 51
United Nations Educational, Scientific and Cultural Organization 110
universal object relationships 66
unthought known 81–82

vagal nerve 142, 151
vicarious introspection 89, 90
video recordings 100–101
Vienna 17, 21–22, 23, 54, 56, 88
Vienna Psychoanalytic Society 49
violence, human propensity for 8; *see also* aggressive impulses

war 66
war neurosis 65
war nurseries 50

well-being, analysts' own 77
White, William Alanson 108
White Institute 111, 112
William Alanson White Psychiatric Foundation 110
Winnicott, Donald 3, 21, 22, 27, 44, 72–78, 96, 97, 118, 127, 128, 136, 143
wisdom 59
wish fulfillment 8, 14, 15
women: Clara Thompson's work on 113; Freud's bias against 113; hysteria 6–7
working alliances 61
working models 128–129
World Health Organization 55, 126
World War I 8, 24, 69, 72, 107
World War II 21, 22–23, 24, 37, 50, 72, 126

Young-Breuhl, E. 22, 49, 50, 51, 64

For Product Safety Concerns and Information please contact our EU
representative GPSR@taylorandfrancis.com
Taylor & Francis Verlag GmbH, Kaufingerstraße 24, 80331 München, Germany

www.ingramcontent.com/pod-product-compliance
Ingram Content Group UK Ltd.
Pitfield, Milton Keynes, MK11 3LW, UK
UKHW020204200926
475702UK00004B/605
* 9 7 8 1 1 3 8 6 0 7 1 2 5 *